"Kimberley Quinlan is a wonderful advocate for self-compassion. Having met her, compassion is something she emanates from her very being. She integrates exposure and response prevention (ERP) and self-compassion in her work with people with obsessive-compulsive disorder (OCD), and is now showing how important and useful self-compassion is for OCD recovery through this book."

—**Stuart Ralph**, child and adolescent counselor and psychotherapist,
   and host of *The OCD Stories* podcast

"Healing becomes possible when we realize we don't have to believe our thoughts. The exercises in this comprehensive and accessible workbook offer those suffering with OCD guidance in meeting mental stories with a patient, forgiving, and wakeful presence. The fruit is a true taste of inner freedom and well-being."

—**Tara Brach**, author of *Radical Acceptance* and *Radical Compassion*

"Reclaiming your life from OCD requires doing some one-eighties. Learning to face—not avoid—your fears. Treating yourself nicely rather than beating yourself up. And you are holding the only book that teaches you how to do both at the same time! This is the guide to learning how to do self-compassionate ERP for OCD, written by one of the most talented and compassionate ERP therapists I know."

—**Shala Nicely, LPC**, author of *Taming OCD, Reclaiming My Life*,
   and *Is Fred in the Refrigerator?*

"If you feel stuck and alone in your struggle against OCD, here's great news. Within you is a storehouse of energy—your compassionate self. With Kimberly Quinlan's workbook, you'll learn to rejuvenate your spirit so that you can push forward into those daunting challenges. On the other side of this effort is the reward: living a life you love."

—**Reid Wilson, PhD**, author of *Stopping the Noise in Your Head*

"*The Self-Compassion Workbook for OCD* is a must-have for both therapists who treat OCD and for those who suffer from OCD. It contains essential, research-based tools to fight OCD while also presenting important and practical self-compassion skills to help sufferers better manage their OCD symptoms. The workbook is friendly, easy to read, and offers concrete examples to follow. I look forward to using this workbook with my clients."

—**Michelle Massi, LMFT**, licensed marriage and family therapist,
    and founder and director of Anxiety Therapy LA

"Years after my diagnosis, the shame, guilt, and self-hatred I had for myself made treatment feel impossible. Much later, I began learning the art of self-compassion. It's been life-altering. Kim's book must live in every clinician and individual's toolbox. This book not only gives the reader the skills to successfully manage OCD and related disorders, but to managing life and all that comes with it."

—**Ethan S. Smith**, national advocate of the International OCD Foundation

The
Self-Compassion
Workbook for OCD

Lean into Your Fear,
Manage Difficult Emotions
& Focus On Recovery

KIMBERLEY QUINLAN, LMFT

New Harbinger Publications, Inc.

Copyright © 2021 by Kimberley Quinlan
New Harbinger Publications, Inc.
5720 Shattuck Avenue
Oakland, CA 94609
www.newharbinger.com

Self-Compassion Break, Affectionate Breathing, Compassionate Friend Meditation, and Giving and Receiving Meditation are from *The Mindful Self-Compassion Workbook*, © 2018 Kristin Neff and Chris Germer. Published by the Guilford Press. Used by Permission.

Cover design by Amy Shoup; Interior design by Michele Waters; Acquired by Tesilya Hanauer

Library of Congress Cataloging-in-Publication Data

Names: Quinlan, Kimberley, author. | Hershfield, Jon, author.
Title: The self-compassion workbook for OCD : lean into your fear, manage difficult emotions, and focus on recovery / Kimberley Quinlan, LMFT, Jon Hershfield.
Description: Oakland : New Harbinger Publication, 2021. | Includes bibliographical references.
Identifiers: LCCN 2021014884 | ISBN 9781684037766 (trade paperback)
Subjects: LCSH: Obsessive-compulsive disorder. | Self-acceptance. | Compassion. | Mindfulness (Psychology)
Classification: LCC RC533 .Q85 2021 | DDC 616.85/227--dc23
LC record available at https://lccn.loc.gov/2021014884

Printed in the United States of America

26   25   24

10   9   8   7   6   5

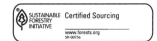

Contents

Foreword

A lot of forewords start with a statement like "I was first introduced to [insert concept here] in …" And I was just about to do that. "I was first introduced to self-compassion in …" 2015? Is that possible? What a strange thing to say. How is it that something so basic and fundamental as being good and kind to yourself never occurred to me on its own? Stranger than that, no one bothered to mention it to me! Did others know and keep it a secret? It certainly wasn't taught in school. And, sorry, Mom and Dad, but I don't recall either of you bringing it up. I had read about it, and of course, I used it with my clients, but to organically use self-compassion for my … um … *self* felt a bit like break dancing or playing a harmonica or riding a unicycle—things I don't know how to do.

Let me tell you a quick story that makes me look really, really lame. I was on a meditation retreat— several days of silence, sitting, walking, eating, and self-compassion training. It can be brutal, this self-compassion stuff. I'm sitting there, trying to be mindful of the noise my brain makes, trying to be nonjudgmental of the constant judgment going through my head. We were doing a RAIN meditation (a technique which Kimberley Quinlan gracefully describes in this book), and it came time for the *N: Nurture*. The teacher invited us to find something to say to ourselves that reflected a genuine permission to feel what was being felt in that moment. This right here is what self-compassion is all about, to look at our pain and say, "I see you feel this—people feel this—you are allowed to be a person who feels this." I waited for the right thought to arise, some mindful ninja warrior thought like "all things are impermanent" or "when you find the Buddha, kill him." I waited and waited and waited. I got bored and stopped looking for the right thought. Then the thought arose in a tone so sweet, it was like a hand just gently landed on my shoulder, so genuine and warm, and so loud I could've sworn it was audible… "It's okay, baby." Laugh all you want, I meant it.

Standing up to adversity, including the adversity of our own mental health challenges, is always hard, but it is so much harder when we disallow ourselves from being people with challenges in the first place. We repeatedly engage in self-criticism and self-punishment, because we are living under the delusion that it works, that it promotes better behavior. It's all based on confusion. We say, "I should know better than to be in this distress" while actively ignoring that our genetics, place of birth, cultural context, and most of our conditioning have nothing to do with us. We think we are bad because we notice vulgar thoughts and disgusting feelings. But what causes us to notice has nothing to do with us. We self-punish because we think it will make better thoughts and feelings arise, but all punishment really does is invite us to be more committed to avoidance. As Kimberley so masterfully lays out in the pages ahead, self-compassion is the path to change. It is the power move in the face of pain. It is the one thing OCD never sees coming.

I met Kimberley around the time I first got licensed as a marriage and family therapist, and she was just starting to earn her clinical hours at the same treatment center. We were fast friends and would have hilarious and meaningful chats about the work we do treating OCD. The way she tells it, I was a bit of a mentor to her. My memory paints a different story of two people learning from each other. It's easy to tell who will make a good OCD therapist, in my opinion. It's not them having OCD, and it's not how much training they've had or whom they studied under. It's the ability to truly understand what the person with OCD feels like. That enables you with the ability to communicate the treatment tools in a language that can be received, while still validating the very real suffering that one endures at the hands of this disorder. It hurts a little, frankly, to really recognize what OCD does to someone from their perspective. Kimberley has always, right from the start, been beautifully pained by her clients' suffering. She is the definition of compassion—full of empathy and the desire to reduce suffering.

I have written extensively about mindfulness for OCD and the challenge has always been to address the "how" of an experiential concept. Mindfulness is not something we *do* or *use*, but is a perspective we take on our experience in the moment. People want to know: *How do I be mindful? What do I actually do?* It can be a bit like telling someone to simply see an optical illusion for what it is. That instruction is not easy to put into a step-by-step manual. Kimberley faces a similar challenge head-on in this book with the concept of self-compassion. *Okay, I'll be self-compassionate. Now what?* This book lays it all out, step by step. But it is about more than simply feeling better. Kimberley masterfully takes the energy of self-compassion and teaches you how to wield it—*weaponize* it, even—against obsessions and compulsions.

Exposure and response prevention (ERP), the most effective treatment we have for OCD, gets a bad rap for being inhumane, torturous, and superficial. It is, in fact, none of the above. It can be empowering, uplifting, and the deepest psychological work you can ever do, tapping into the core of your humanity. It is hard, of course, but it is never in the service of cruelty or pain for pain's sake. At the core of ERP is always self-compassion. It's about acknowledging, *Hey, this is hard, and compulsions teach the brain that you can't handle it. Let's try something else. Let's put ourselves in situations in which we feel the urge to do compulsions, and let's show the brain how much faith we have in its ability to choose a different path.*

At the end of the day, much of what keeps us trapped in the obsessive-compulsive cycle is how we believe we'll treat ourselves if our fears were to come true. If the engrained belief is that we'll be cruel toward ourselves, abusive and exclusively self-punitive, then we will always argue in favor of avoidance. But if, instead, our assumption were to be that we'd cope somehow, that we'd hold ourselves in the same kindness we would offer someone we cared about, that we deserve better than what OCD tells us, it's possible a lot of our compulsions would seem superfluous. Uncertainty can feel like a scary, winding path through a forest at night, but self-compassion can be the hand you hold along the way. Just past this clearing, around the bend, a few more steps, there is hope. We got this.

—Jon Hershfield, MFT, The Center for OCD and Anxiety at Sheppard Pratt

Introduction

Welcome to *The Self-Compassion Workbook for OCD: A Mindful and Compassionate Approach to Help You Manage Difficult Emotions, Lean into Your Fear, and Focus on Recovery.*

The Purpose of This Book

For the last decade, I have had the pleasure of specializing in the treatment of obsessive-compulsive disorder (OCD) and OCD-related conditions. It has been one of the greatest joys in my life to help people with OCD change the way they respond to anxiety and teach them how to live a life where anxiety doesn't make their decisions.

When I started my internship as a marriage and family therapist and OCD specialist, I was eager to help my patients with OCD manage their obsessions and compulsions. However, I quickly realized that they needed help with more than their obsessions and compulsions. What I observed was that these wonderfully kind, smart, hilarious, and talented human beings were also being tormented, day in and day out, by a deep sense of guilt, shame, and humiliation. They reported spending an exorbitant amount of time criticizing and punishing themselves for the intrusive thoughts, feelings, sensations, images, and urges they experienced and for the compulsive behaviors they performed to remove the anxiety and uncertainty that they felt.

As each patient told me their OCD story, I could not help but feel deeply connected with them, as I had previously found myself in a similar situation. When I had battled an eating disorder, I spent hours every day mentally and physically calculating every single calorie I had eaten and compulsively exercising to remove the anxiety and uncertainty that tormented me. I engaged in relentless negative self-talk, self-doubt, and self-punishment, believing that is what I deserved and hoping that would keep me in line.

During my treatment, I learned the importance of having a strong self-compassion practice, and to this day, I have found self-compassion to be the cornerstone of my long-term recovery. I started teaching my clients and patients with OCD every self-compassion tool I knew, and right before my eyes, I could see a transformation that still brings me to tears. People who treated themselves in ways they would never dream of treating even their worst enemy became people who treated themselves with kindness, loyalty, and acceptance.

I have made it my mission to teach self-compassion and mindfulness skills to those who struggle with anxiety. I produce a podcast, Your Anxiety Toolkit Podcast, on which I interview world-renowned self-compassion researchers and mindfulness teachers, such as Paul Gilbert, Kristin Neff, Tara Brach, Dennis Tirch, and Steven Hayes, discussing how to apply their research and practices to meet the needs of those with OCD. I also interview and pick the brains of some of the leading and most innovative clinicians and researchers in the field, such as Reid Wilson, Jon Hershfield, Shala Nicely, David Burns, Jonathon Grayson, Stuart Ralph, and Patrick McGrath, discussing what they feel to be the most effective tools and treatment practices for OCD. This workbook is jam-packed with the science-based treatment tools and self-compassion practices that have enriched my life and the lives of my clients with OCD. I have no doubt that they will help you take back your life from OCD and learn to treat yourself with the love, compassion, and respect that you deserve.

The Science Behind Self-Compassion

Fortunately, we now have much research to prove the widespread benefits of practicing self-compassion. The practice of self-compassion is associated with lower levels of anxiety, depression, and rumination and higher levels of motivation, resulting in general improvements in well-being (Warren et al. 2016). Scientific findings have also identified that the imagery of receiving compassion decreases the excretion of cortisol, the stress hormone responsible for our bodies' fight-or-flight response (Rockliff et al. 2008).

Research also shows how beneficial self-compassion can be for those with OCD. The practice of self-compassion reduces OCD severity and allows the person with OCD to better manage their feelings of shame, guilt, frustration, low self-worth, and inadequacy (Wetterneck et al. 2013). Wetterneck and his collogues also found that self-compassion reduces the rates of treatment drop-out. This research is ground breaking and sheds light on the common hurdles faced by those in OCD treatment. Lastly, researchers have found that the practice of self-compassion aids in people's ability to regulate their emotions and is related to high levels of overall positive mental health (Trompetter et al. 2016). Incredible, right?

But First, Let's Clear One Thing Up!

Before we move forward, let me clarify a couple of important things. Self-compassion is *not* flowers and unicorns. It does not involve simply giving yourself compliments and permission to run away from the many fears and struggles you experience. The practice of self-compassion involves a deep commitment to not only treating yourself with loving kindness, tenderness, and self-respect, but also standing up to fear and being intentional about no longer allowing fear to make your choices and rule your life. Self-compassion encompasses the deep wish for your own wellness and happiness. Self-compassion is the practice of honoring and tenderly making space for the discomfort you experience instead of pushing it away. Self-compassion is warm, yet fierce.

What to Expect

Throughout this workbook, I will ask you to participate in many practical exercises, meditations, and self-reflections. I will repetitively convey how important it is that you make a commitment to yourself to practice these skills on a daily basis. Your long-term recovery from OCD really depends on your willingness to keep practicing, even when things get hard. In fact, the more challenging things are and the more you are struggling, the more you will benefit by leaning into these tools and practices.

Based on the fact that you have chosen to keep reading, I am confident that you are committed to living a more compassionate life with OCD. As we move together through this workbook, I will provide you with four case studies to help you conceptualize how to implement the tools included in this workbook and also understand the common roadblocks to practicing self-compassion and a tool called "exposure and response prevention" (ERP). In a moment, I am going to introduce you to the people in these case studies, Alex, Tanya, Todd, and Simone. They all have OCD and have learned that they, too, are deserving of kindness, tenderness, and self-respect. These case studies are based on actual patients and clients I have treated, but to protect their confidentiality, their names and characteristics have been altered. Together, Alex, Tanya, Todd, Simone, and I are going to be right by your side as you too learn how to manage your obsessions and compulsions and live a more compassionate and empowered life.

— Meet Alex!

One morning, Alex, a twenty-seven-year-old elementary school teacher, woke up to the breaking news announcing that a teacher from a nearby school district was arrested for sexually and physically assaulting seven students. Alex was horrified. Within a few minutes of hearing this news, Alex was hit with an onslaught of anxiety. *What if I hurt one of my students? Could I? Do I want to? What if I want to? Is it possible that I might secretly enjoy these thoughts? Why would I even think this? What if I go to jail? What if...?* These thoughts went on and on and on.

For months following, Alex spent hundreds of hours trying to solve whether he was capable of harming his students. Even when Alex could form some kind of reassurance that he would never perform such an act, it would not be long until he was hit with another terrorizing wave of fear and uncertainty. When I met Alex, he had quit his job, because his students made him so anxious that he could not get through a class without panicking. Alex spent all day berating himself for his thoughts and feelings, and his inability to control them.

⌐ Meet Tanya!

Tanya is a thirty-nine-year-old design executive for a fashion magazine. Tanya has relationship OCD and sexual orientation OCD. Tanya came out as a lesbian when she was seventeen years old, and her family lovingly supported her. Three years ago, Tanya and her then girlfriend, Julie, got engaged. But in this wonderful celebratory time of her life, she quickly became overwhelmed with intrusive thoughts and uncertainty about whether she was gay or straight. For months leading up to her wedding, Tanya could not help but spend every waking hour trying to figure out if she was gay or straight and was repetitively bombarded with intrusive images of herself having sex with men. The thing that scared her the most was that sometimes she felt aroused by these images. Tanya repetitively checked to see if she was aroused or attracted to her partner and spent many evenings secretly watching pornography and television shows with lesbian characters to reassure herself that she was, in fact, attracted to women.

Tanya also experienced relationship obsessions in which she questioned if her love for Julie was "pure" or "deep enough." No matter how hard she tried, Tanya could not be certain if Julie was "the one." Tanya felt tremendous guilt and shame about her sexual orientation obsessions and her inability to be certain about her love for Julie. Over time, Tanya became painfully self-critical, judging herself harshly for the thoughts she was having, and she would scold herself for having these struggles.

⌐ Meet Todd!

Todd, seventeen years old, is a senior in high school and has already been awarded a scholarship to a top college to play basketball. When he was fourteen, Todd was diagnosed with "not just right" obsessions and compulsions, commonly known as "just right OCD." Todd is a smart, driven young man who would literally not allow himself to rest until he "felt" he had completed tasks perfectly or did so in a "just right" way. Todd has engaged in these behaviors since he was a young boy, but recently Todd and his parents had noticed that his compulsive need for things to be perfect was now getting in the way of his well-being and impacting the entire family. Todd was having multiple panic attacks per day, his grades were starting to drop, he was missing basketball trainings, and he was beginning to experience severe stomachaches at night.

Todd felt like he had to move objects back and forth, or he would have to count in multiples of two or four until it felt just right. Todd also washed his hands repetitively until his hands "felt clean." He sometimes had to wash his hands over a hundred times. He would also yell and sometimes scream cruel and hateful words toward himself until he was able to get things feeling right. Todd would also sometimes repetitively hit himself when he could not get an object in the right position. When I met Todd, he said he felt hopeless and completely exhausted, leaving him and his parents heartbroken.

— Meet Simone!

Simone, a pharmacist, came to see me after being put on medical leave. Simone loved her job and was devastated that she had to take time off to get treatment for her OCD. Simone had recently been diagnosed with scrupulosity and moral OCD by her psychiatrist. Simone hated herself for not being able to control her thoughts and compulsive behaviors and was still questioning her diagnosis of OCD. One of the most essential roles in Simone's job was filling prescriptions for her customers. When Simone checked that the dose and quantity of the pills were correct, she would have intrusive thoughts about possibly adding in other serious, deadly medications to the patient's bottle. These thoughts went completely against Simone's values and morals, but she could not shake the fear that she was capable of such an act. Simone would "get stuck"—checking and rechecking the pill bottles—and her boss and coworkers would get annoyed with her, because she would get behind with her prescription orders. Once Simone left work for the day, she would mentally go over the steps she had taken with each patient's prescription and would try to remember if she had either made a mistake or even purposely tampered with the doses. Each morning, Simone would pray to God, asking to be forgiven for her sins, even though she was not sure if she had sinned or not. Simone would also get stuck during prayer, repetitively asking God to make sure she never mixes medications or doses. Simone would call herself horrible names and tell herself that she deserves to go to hell for what she has done. Simone very much valued her Christianity, so telling herself that this is what she deserved showed how hard Simone was on herself for the thoughts she was having and the uncertainty she felt.

How This Book Is Organized

This workbook is organized into three parts. Part 1 will teach you about the cycle of OCD and how self-criticism, self-blame, and self-punishment only reinforce this cycle. You will also learn the core self-compassion concepts and practices you will need for your long-term recovery and the common roadblocks that those with OCD experience. Part 2 will show you how to apply self-compassion and mindfulness through each and every step of exposure and response prevention. You will create your own Self-Compassionate Exposure and Response Prevention plan and practice ERP using self-compassion as your superpower. Lastly, part 3 will address what long-term recovery looks like and, finally, help you to address the trauma, grief, and loss associated with having OCD.

There is a website for this book (http://www.newharbinger.com/47766), where you can find copies of some exercises to download and print, as well as some audio recordings of meditations that I have made.

Before we get started, I want to thank you for trusting me to be on this journey with you. I am well aware that you had many great options for OCD workbooks to choose from. I am so grateful for the opportunity to be a part of your self-compassion journey. You deserve nothing but kindness and respect. I hope you learn to become your own best friend and an unconditional source of support throughout your recovery.

PART ONE

From Self-Criticism to Self-Compassion

Hello, my friend,

This is the first of a number of letters throughout this workbook. Consider each letter a personal note from me to you to support and guide you as you move through the different stages of your recovery. May each and every letter provide you with compassion, validation, and inspiration.

Three things in human life are important.

The first is to be kind.

The second is to be kind.

And the third is to be kind.

—Henry James

Let's translate that, shall we? When you have anxiety, be kind to yourself. When you have an obsession, be kind to yourself. When you face your fears, be kind to yourself. When you are feeling strong emotions, be kind to yourself. When you feel like you are failing, be kind to yourself. The more you suffer, the more self-compassion you deserve.

I wholeheartedly believe in you,

Kimberley

CHAPTER 1

Understanding Obsessive-Compulsive Disorder

Obsessive-compulsive disorder (OCD) is a brain-based mental health disorder that involves obsessions and compulsions. An *obsession* is an unwanted, intrusive thought, feeling, sensation, or urge that is repetitive and induces a significant degree of anxiety, uncertainty, doubt, or disgust. *Compulsions* are both physical and mental behaviors that are done to reduce or remove anxiety, uncertainty, or another form of discomfort. These obsessions and compulsions are exhausting and can significantly impair daily functioning and quality of life.

When defining OCD, it is just as important to clearly address what it is *not*. Unfortunately, our society still fails to understand that OCD is not a quirky personality trait and that the term "OCD" should not be used as an adjective, such as "I am so OCD!" Having OCD does not involve enthusiastically arranging the contents of your kitchen cupboards or stacking your cookies in a perfect pattern in the cookie jar. Having OCD is not an experience you joke about with your friends or coworkers. Having OCD is not simply being superstitious and knocking on wood to ward off misfortune or bring good luck. While these examples can look similar to the presentation of OCD, the difference is that people with OCD find their obsessions and compulsions incredibly painful, humiliating, and exhausting. While there is nothing to be ashamed of by having obsessive-compulsive disorder, it is not something anyone would ever ask for or wear as a badge of honor. In fact, many people with OCD say that they would never wish OCD on even their worst enemy.

To be officially diagnosed with OCD, you need to be formally assessed by a trained mental health provider or medical doctor and fulfill specific diagnostic criteria. If you are interested in finding a specialized OCD provider, check the therapist directory at the International OCD Foundation's website (https://iocdf.org), or you can do an internet search to see if there is a provider in your area. If you do not have access to such providers, you may use the information listed above as a general guide. However, please remember that this workbook cannot replace a mental health or medical provider's assessment and treatment.

Before you learn the specific science-based tools to manage your OCD, it is essential that you first understand the mechanics of obsessive-compulsive disorder. Just as with any problem or roadblock, understanding the mechanisms of the problem is crucial before you can begin crafting a solution. In this chapter, you will learn to conceptualize and understand your OCD using the obsessive-compulsive cycle (commonly called the O-C cycle). Using this conceptualization, you will learn what behaviors keep the cycle going and how to break your own O-C cycle using self-compassion and the gold standard treatment of OCD, exposure and response prevention (ERP). In addition, once you understand the biological and physiological factors involved in OCD, you will come to recognize that having OCD was never your fault and that if you put any human being in your exact situation, they would respond in exactly the way you have in the past. Lastly, my wish is that this chapter (with Alex as your case study) will help you recognize that your obsessions and compulsions are in no way a reflection of your intelligence, worth, or strength and that criticizing yourself makes the O-C cycle stronger and slows down recovery.

Every OCD Story Starts with an Obsession

Your first experience with having OCD began the moment you experienced your first obsession. This obsession presented itself in the form of a repetitive, intrusive, and unwanted thought, image, feeling, sensation, or urge. Your obsessions maybe presented as a "what if?" thought, an image of an unwanted event, a sensation or feeling that raised a sense of alarm, or an urge to perform some kind of action that concerned you.

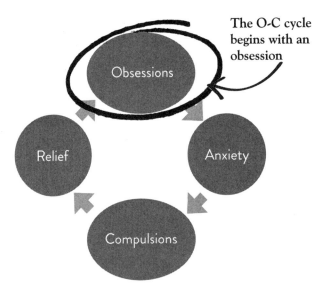

Figure 1. Every OCD Story Starts with an Obsession

Subtypes of Obsessive-Compulsive Disorder

While every person with OCD has their own unique set of intrusive thoughts, images, sensations, feelings, and urges, researchers and mental health clinicians often arrange the most common obsessions into specific categories or groups, called OCD subtypes. These obsession subtypes are categorized into groups for research purposes and also to create effective and streamlined treatment plans. Many people with OCD report that these OCD subtypes have also helped them feel less alone, recognizing that others are struggling with obsessions with similar content.

I have outlined the most common subtypes below for your reference. Using the check boxes provided, place a check mark next to any subtypes that resonate with your experience. Please remember that every person's OCD looks different, even within the subtype categories. Also, please do not be alarmed if your specific obsessions are not included. I have kept the list as concise as possible for ease of use. You will have an opportunity to create a comprehensive list of your specific obsessions and compulsions later in this workbook.

- ☐ *Contamination OCD.* The fear and uncertainty that germs, chemicals, and other contaminants will make one sick or even terminally ill. Contamination OCD also includes obsessions of repulsion and disgust.

- ☐ *Symmetry OCD.* The anxiety and discomfort that objects are not lined up correctly, are asymmetrical, or are not in a particular pattern.

- ☐ *Sexual Orientation OCD.* Fear and uncertainty surrounding one's sexual orientation. In the past, this obsession was commonly called "homosexual OCD" (HOCD). But because obsessions can become focused on any sexual orientation, we now use the inclusive term "sexual orientation OCD," because a person of any sexual orientation can struggle with the uncertainty of having or developing a different orientation. Obsessions surrounding one's gender identity are also common.

- ☐ *Just Right OCD.* The fear and discomfort related to experiencing a "not right" feeling. This subtype of OCD can be "fixed" (with the individual always feeling that things need to be a precise and particular way) or ever-changing (with the individual's feelings of "rightness" changing, depending on what feels "right" at that moment).

- ☐ *Harm OCD.* The fear and uncertainty around whether one could or did, accidentally or intentionally, hurt others or oneself.

- ☐ *Pedophilia OCD (commonly known as POCD).* The fear and uncertainty related to being or becoming a pedophile. Common POCD obsessions include fears related to possibly being aroused by or attracted to a minor or the fear of intentionally or unintentionally having performed a sexual behavior with a minor in the past or doing so in the future.

- ☐ *Perinatal OCD.* The uncertainty and fear of harming one's newborn baby or child, either physically or sexually. Perinatal OCD is a subtype of OCD that can be experienced by both female and male primary caretakers, not just the person who delivered the baby.

- ☐ *Scrupulosity or Moral OCD.* The fear and uncertainty about possibly offending one's religious figure (such as God), possibly performing a behavior that doesn't align with one's morals or religion, or the fear of not achieving a desired afterlife.

☐ *Relationship OCD (commonly known as ROCD).* The uncertainty and fear related to knowing if one's partner is "the one" or if their love for their partner is "pure" or "right." Relationship obsessions can also focus on a partner's specific body part or their partner's history.

☐ *Emotional Contamination OCD.* The uncertainty and fear that contact with a person, object, or place will alter them psychologically. Emotional contamination OCD also involves the fear that the contaminated person's "essence" will be transferred onto the person with OCD.

☐ *Existential OCD.* The fear and uncertainty about the true purpose or meaning of one's life.

☐ *Obsessing about Obsessing.* The uncertainty and fear that one will never be able to stop obsessing or having anxiety and intrusive thoughts. This OCD subtype also involves the uncertainty related to whether they are engaging in treatment correctly or will recover from OCD.

☐ *Sensorimotor or Hyper-Awareness OCD.* The uncertainty and fear that one will never stop noticing a sensation or feeling (breath, eyes, blinking, hands tingling, a specific side of their body or body part, itches, and so on).

☐ *Hyper-Responsibility OCD.* The uncertainty and fear of being responsible for a tragic event, other people's feelings or well-being.

☐ *Health Anxiety.* The uncertainty and fear of having or developing a severe or terminal illness. Health anxiety obsessions can also focus on the health of a loved one, such as a child or partner.

☐ *Perfectionism.* The uncertainty and fear related to not being perfect. This doesn't necessarily mean the person with perfectionism needs everything to be perfect. Perfectionism can target one area of one's life or can spread to every aspect of one's life.

Alex   For Alex, a teacher who loves helping young people learn, the onset of his obsessions began when he saw the news and had the thought, *What if I want to kill my students?* This intrusive thought was accompanied with an intrusive urge that rose inside him. This aggressive urge made him feel like he could lose control and go on a killing spree. Alex reported that his first obsession was different from any other thought he had ever had, and it felt like something in his brain "broke."

Alex knew that he was not the type of person who would want to harm anyone, especially his students. However, these thoughts brought on a barrage of painful self-criticisms. Alex was repulsed by his thoughts. Instead of acknowledging that everyone has these kinds of thoughts sometimes, Alex displaced blame onto himself. Alex labeled himself as "bad" and "disgusting," and his relationship with himself went from being mostly kind and supportive to hateful and self-punishing.

Reflection

How have your specific obsessions changed the way you view yourself? Do you treat yourself differently when you have these obsessions?

_____

_____

_____

_____

Use the space below to identify the critical words or statements you use toward yourself when you experience intrusive thoughts, images, sensations, feelings, or urges. As you reflect, be careful not to engage in this self-criticism. Try to just write them down and move on to the next question.

_____

_____

_____

_____

How does it make you feel when you see the words written in front of you?

_____

_____

_____

_____

The Obsession Leads to Anxiety and Uncertainty

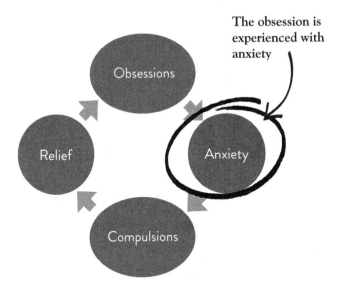

Figure 2. An Obsession Leads to Anxiety and Uncertainty

Okay, folks! Let's geek out a little and go into some detail about the science of your brain. Understanding what is actually happening in your brain can be tremendously helpful, as it gives you insight into why you have such an overwhelming experience of anxiety and why anxiety sometimes feels so uncontrollable. Understanding these processes can also help your self-compassion practice, as it can help you to see that the thoughts, feelings, images, sensations, and urges you experience are not your fault and simply a glitch in the neurological system.

Deep in your brain is an almond-shaped structure called the amygdala, which contains a set of neurons that detect danger. When your amygdala interprets a thought, feeling, sensation, or urge as dangerous, it immediately begins a process that results in chemicals and hormones being released throughout your body to protect you from the potential threat. Those chemicals and hormones are responsible for your physical experience of anxiety, such as an increased heart rate, a spinning head, stomach discomfort, sweating, or chest pain, just to name a few.

This physiological process is called the fight-or-flight-or-freeze response (FFF for short) and is crucial for our survival. For example, when your brain interprets danger, the FFF response may signal the release of adrenaline, giving you a surge of aggression and strength to fight off the threat. This is the *fight* response in action. Alternatively, you may also notice that your heart rate and breathing patterns increase rapidly. This is an example of the *flight* response, preparing you to run away from the danger. The flight response may also signal for the release of hormones such as cortisol, which prompts your body to eliminate any excess weight in the bowel and bladder to make it easier for you to run away. This explains why you might need to go to the restroom right away when an obsession triggers you.

There will be times where fighting or running away (fight or flight) is not appropriate. For instance, if you were in close proximity to a snake, lion, or another aggressive beast, but the animal hadn't noticed you, your body might instead go into a *freeze* mode. In this case, your nervous system pumps the neurological "brakes" so that you freeze and stand completely still until the beast or perceived danger passes without harming you.

Now, there are times when your brain sets off the alarm bells even when there is no imminent threat. The evolution of the human brain has resulted in an instinctive response to danger, which prepares us for the fight, flight, or freeze, even when faced with an inkling of *possibility* for danger. As a result, our brains send out a danger signal and the FFF response, *just in case!* This "just in case" function can cause you to feel as if everything and anything is dangerous or potentially harmful.

We also have scientific research that shows that there are key differences in the brains of those with OCD that can also help us understand why your thoughts, feelings, sensations, images, and urges feel so strong. Brain scans have shown that the amygdala of someone with OCD is hypersensitive to danger and generates a rapid firing of danger signals, causing the person with OCD to experience a series of false alarms (Simon et al. 2014).

Why Can't I Stop the Obsessions?

Alex   During Alex's first session, when I was educating him on how we plan to break the O-C cycle, he asked me a question that almost every single client has asked me at some point during treatment. "But, Kimberley, can't you just teach me how to stop the obsessions?"

Let's answer this question by doing a little activity.

The Green Apple Exercise

If you can, set a timer for three minutes. During this time, I would like you to do your best to *not* think about a green apple. Every time you accidentally think about a green apple, please mark one tally on the line below. Don't worry about how many tally marks you have during the three minutes. Just do your best to *not* think about that apple. Ready, set, go!

_____

Reflection

Okay, how did that go? What did you assume would happen? How many tally marks did you get? Were you surprised by this exercise?

_____

_____

_____

_____

_____

I am guessing that as you tried to suppress the thought about a green apple, you observed an increase in the intensity and frequency of that thought. This phenomenon is called the "ironic rebound effect" (Wegner et al. 1987). This is because the very act of trying *not* to think about something results in you actually thinking about the thing even more. The act of not thinking about something is actually thinking about it. This is exactly what happens when you try not to think about your obsession.

Interestingly, studies have found that when people with OCD attempted to suppress their thoughts, they reported almost double the tally marks of non-anxious and generally anxious participants (Tolin et al. 2000). These scientific findings suggests that people with OCD have deficits in the cognitive "brakes," resulting in repetitive, intrusive thoughts, feelings, sensations, urges, and images.

Whom Do You Blame?

Alex   In Alex's second session with me, he shared that he was so angry with and ashamed of his "stupid brain." Between sessions, Alex decided to share his experience with OCD with his best friend, Jeff, who worked as a dance instructor. Alex was shocked to hear that Jeff had experienced similar thoughts about his students in the past, but that Jeff wasn't worried about them and didn't give these thoughts any of his time. After learning this, Alex started comparing himself negatively, painfully blaming his brain for creating this situation he was in. Alex would make sarcastic jokes about how his brain was "messed up" for setting off his FFF response, resulting in high degrees of anxiety, while Jeff's brain simply moved on.

Alex and I explored the idea of not blaming himself for his OCD or for how his brain responds to these thoughts. Instead, he worked to recognize that having OCD was no one's fault. Alex set the intention of validating himself when he had intrusive thoughts, telling himself, *I am noticing that my brain has set off the alarm again. Because I now understand my brain, it makes sense that this is scary for me.* Alex also practiced recognizing that some people's brains are genetically set up to have obsessions and compulsions. Given that his grandmother also had OCD, Alex worked to not attribute blame to himself or his grandmother.

Reflection

Whom do you blame for your obsessions and compulsions? Do you condemn your brain for the way it functions? What words have you previously used to describe your brain and the way your brain functions?

_____

_____

_____

_____

_____

What can you now tell yourself?

_____

_____

_____

_____

_____

_____

Anxiety Leads to a Compulsion

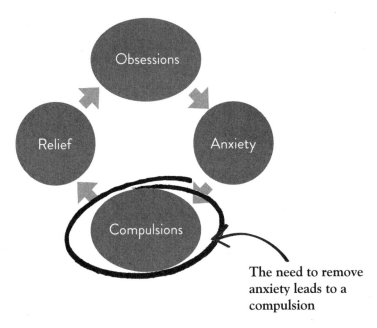

The need to remove anxiety leads to a compulsion

Figure 3. Anxiety Leads to a Compulsion

Naturally, humans will go to any length to avoid discomfort, especially if it is in the form of anxiety or uncertainty. Whether your anxiety is mild, moderate, or high, you will intuitively try to move away from it. In the psychology field, we often call the act of moving away from discomfort or perceived danger a "safety behavior"—an internal or external action performed in an effort to protect oneself from danger or help cope with a stressful or dangerous situation. Throughout this workbook, you will see me use the terms "safety-seeking behaviors" and "compulsions" interchangeably.

Alex   When Alex wakes up in the morning, he is hit with a barrage of intrusive thoughts about harming his students. The anxiety and uncertainty are so painful that Alex engages in a series of reassurance-seeking behaviors and hours of mental rumination to try to figure out if he is capable of doing such an act. Alex reports that he feels like he has no control of these safety-seeking behaviors: "I cannot stop no matter how hard I try."

Once again, we can rely on science to help us understand why Alex and other people with OCD struggle with controlling their compulsive behaviors. Brain scans of people with OCD have shown that the part of the brain that processes errors is overactive (Norman et al. 2019). This study also reported that the part of the brain that would normally pump the breaks on safety-seeking behaviors is impaired, explaining the difficulty that people with OCD have resisting compulsions. Hopefully, these findings will help you understand why you (like Alex) struggle to stop yourself from engaging in compulsive behaviors. Getting stuck doing compulsions is not a reflection of a lack of willpower, work ethic, or intelligence.

Spoiler Alert!

Despite these small differences in your brain, there is an abundance of evidence-based skills and practices that can help you reduce and even eliminate your safety-seeking compulsions. In fact, you will learn these exact skills and practices here in this workbook!

Common Compulsions Within OCD Subtypes

In the space below, I have listed some of the most common compulsions for each subtype covered earlier in this chapter. Once again, please note that this is not an exhaustive list and may not include your specific compulsions. In chapter 5, you will prepare a thorough inventory of your obsessions and compulsions. For now, use this list as a reference to help you understand the common compulsions involved in the O-C cycle.

- ☐ *Contamination OCD.* Hand washing; the use of antibacterial products; avoidance of feared substances, objects, or people; requiring or asking family members to perform compulsions for them; and mental rumination.

- ☐ *Symmetry OCD.* Physically or mentally moving or realigning objects, avoiding objects or scenarios where objects may need realigning, and asking for or requiring family members to place objects in a particular way.

- ☐ *Sexual Orientation OCD.* Avoidance of any objects or people who trigger their obsession, mental rumination in an attempt to resolve the uncertainty about one's sexual preference, online reassurance seeking, repetitively questioning if OCD is the correct diagnosis, mentally checking oneself for arousal or sexual preference, intercourse and masturbation as a form of reassurance, and avoidance of pleasure of any kind. Obsessions surrounding one's gender identity is also a common OCD theme and involves similar compulsions.

- ☐ *Just Right OCD.* Repetitively doing *any* action until the "just right" feeling is achieved. This might consist of repetitively moving objects, repetitively walking through doors, repetitively cleaning or touching an item, and so forth. Compulsions also include avoiding events or places, numbers, colors, or words that result in the "not right" feeling, mentally attempting to attain a "just right" feeling, and asking others to change or maintain their behaviors to achieve or maintain the "just right" feeling.

- ☐ *Harm OCD.* Avoidance of loved ones in fear of harming them, avoidance of objects that could cause harm (knives, cars, sharp objects), asking for reassurance to prove one did not hurt another person or is not capable of harming others, mental rumination to find certainty about the intentions of these thoughts, and repetitive questioning if the diagnosis of OCD is correct.

☐ *Pedophilia OCD (POCD)*. Avoidance of children, schools, or daycare centers, or avoiding specific interactions with children (diaper changes, bath time, etc.); mental review; rumination in the hope to achieve certainty about the intentions behind one's thoughts, feelings, images, sensations, and urges; mentally or physically checking for arousal; seeking reassurance from loved ones or the internet to prove one is not a pedophile; and repetitively questioning if OCD is the correct diagnosis.

☐ *Perinatal OCD*. Avoidance of one's baby or child; repetitive reassurance seeking from loved ones and from the internet; mental rumination to find certainty about the intentions of one's thoughts, images, feelings, sensations, and urges; and repetitively questioning if OCD is the correct diagnosis.

☐ *Scrupulosity or Moral OCD*. Repetitive and ritualized prayer; avoidance of blasphemous thoughts and images; avoidance of or excessive attendance of religious events, locations, and people; repetitive and ritualized learning of religious texts; and mental rumination about one's past religious or spiritual behaviors.

☐ *Relationship OCD (ROCD)*. Mentally scrutinizing one's satisfaction with or love for one's partner, comparing of one's own relationship to other people's relationships, confessing obsessions to one's partner, avoiding relationships altogether, asking the partner to change their behaviors or physical attributes, and repetitively breaking up with partners due to the presence of uncertainty.

☐ *Emotional Contamination OCD*. Avoidance of feared person, object, or place; mental rumination of recent exposure to a feared person or object; mental review of upcoming events; and physical or mental neutralization of intrusive thoughts, image, feelings, sensations, or urges.

☐ *Existential OCD*. Mental rumination and repetitive research about the purpose and meaning of life, reassurance-seeking with philosophy scholars or religious or spiritual leaders, avoidance of triggers that debunk their current conceptualization of the meaning of life.

☐ *Obsessing about Obsessing*. Avoidance of anything that may trigger fear, uncertainty, or doubt; repetitive checking to see if they are obsessing or experiencing anxiety; excessive research on treatment and treatment methods; thought suppression; mentally checking anxiety levels; and compulsive treatment seeking.

☐ *Sensorimotor or Hyper-Awareness OCD*. Mental rumination over the sensation or how to get rid of the sensation, avoidance of behaviors that increase the awareness of uncomfortable sensations, repetitive checking to see if they are aware of the sensation.

☐ *Hyper-responsibility OCD.* Repetitively checking objects (if stoves are turned off, doors are locked, candles and matches are out, no one was hurt, and so on), mentally reviewing if someone was hurt, seeking reassurance that no one was physically or emotionally hurt, apologizing for actions that do not require an apology, and tending to "possible" dangers that are not a real, imminent threat.

☐ *Health Anxiety.* Checking one's body for illness, taking one's temperature repetitively, seeking medical advice frequently, searching the internet for symptoms, reassurance seeking, mental rumination, self-punishment, and mental review.

☐ *Perfectionism.* Checking for perfectionism, redoing activities until they are perfect, mental rumination, reassurance seeking, and self-punishment.

Alex   "Why do some people have intrusive thoughts about contamination or another OCD subtype while I have thoughts about killing people or sexually harming them? This must mean something about me. What does having these specific obsessions mean about my character?"

We don't quite know why one person has one obsession and others have another or why some have multiple different obsessions at once. What we do know is that people tend to have obsessions about the things they value the most. Alex deeply cares about his students, so it makes sense that his OCD would target the things he is passionate about. Similarly, a new mother might have intrusive thoughts about harming the child she loves more than she ever imagined. A student, like Todd, who highly values his academics, is likely to have obsessions about perfectionism in his studies. A partner, like Tanya, who deeply loves her significant other, might develop relationship obsessions, for example. Or a pharmacist, like Simone, who deeply cares about being a good employee and about helping her patients might have obsessions about her own morals and ethics.

Compulsions Lead to Relief (Well, Sort Of!)

Usually, a person with OCD will perform a compulsion until they achieve some kind of relief. It might be a relief from anxiety, uncertainty, doubt, disgust, or some other form of discomfort. The relief from compulsions might come quite quickly, in a matter of seconds, or it could take hours of engaging in compulsive behaviors to find relief.

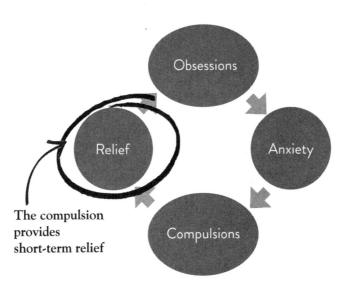

The compulsion
provides
short-term relief

Figure 4. Compulsions Bring Relief

Relief Reinforces the Obsessions ... and the Cycle Continues!

When you perform a compulsive behavior to reduce or remove anxiety, you will likely perceive the behavior to be "effective," because it does provide relief by removing your experience of uncertainty, anxiety, and doubt. This is what we call "negative reinforcement." Because the compulsion provided relief in the past, you will naturally be inclined to engage in the same behavior when the intrusive thoughts returns.

In addition, because compulsions provide short-term relief from anxiety, they reinforce the obsession's perceived validity. Each time you respond to an obsession with a compulsion, you confirm the belief that the fear is "dangerous" and repetitively set off the FFF response. Ironically, when you perform a compulsion, you are also more likely to experience the return of that obsession, because the compulsion is a reminder of the obsession itself.

What is not shown in the O-C cycle diagrams above is that when your obsession returns, you are highly likely to try adding another compulsive behavior to prevent the obsession from returning once and for all. Before too long, this pattern solidifies as a behavioral pattern, and the obsessive-compulsive cycle slowly takes over your life, sometimes impairing your ability to function in any of your daily activities. In conclusion, while compulsions may "work" in that they reduce short-term discomfort, they definitely do not "work" at relieving long-term discomfort. Compulsions always result in reinforcing your obsessions and leave you feeling more and more out of control and disempowered.

Once again, I hope that knowing how human behavior is reinforced can help you understand why it becomes easy to get stuck in an obsessive-compulsive cycle. Your intrusive thoughts and compulsive behaviors are the result of a combination of genetics, human biology, and learned behavior, and this is *not your fault!*

Reflection

How have you judged yourself for your compulsions in the past?

_____

Now that you understand the mechanics of your O-C cycle, what could you tell yourself when you notice you are being judgmental and self-critical of yourself for engaging in compulsions?

_____

_____

_____

Let's Break the Cycle!

To stop the O-C cycle from going around and around, you need to intervene at one of the four stages of the cycle. We already know that you cannot control or stop your obsessions, and you now understand that you are unable to stop your brain from sending out signals of danger and anxiety to the rest of your body. We also recognize that engaging in compulsions provides only short-term relief and that trying to do more and more compulsions only reinforces the return of obsessions.

To break this obsessive-compulsive cycle, we will intervene right before doing a compulsion by employing the gold-standard treatment for OCD, exposure and response prevention (ERP). Instead of trying to find a sense of relief, you are going to practice allowing your intrusive thoughts, feelings, sensations, and urges to occur (or have them purposely) and willingly tolerate the anxiety as it rises and falls on its own. Our goal, together, is to lean into the discomfort of anxiety and uncertainty and work to reduce and remove compulsive safety-seeking behaviors. I understand that this is more easily said than done. However, I have had the pleasure of seeing many, many individuals take their lives back from OCD using this method, *and you can too!* Are you ready to break the cycle?

How Self-Criticism and Self-Punishment Reinforce the O-C Cycle

You may have noticed from your written reflections throughout this chapter how much shame and self-criticism impact your psychological wellness. Not only does the shame and self-criticism increase your anxiety, causing you to feel more distress, but they also increase your urgency to engage in compulsive behaviors. More on this in just a sec!

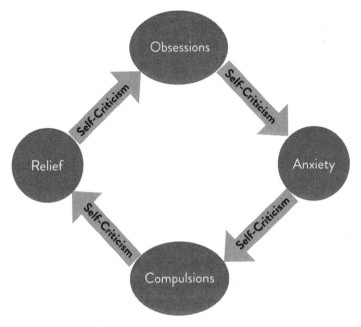

Figure 5. Self-Criticism Strengthens the Cycle

At every stage of the O-C cycle, shame and self-criticism reinforce your obsessions and compulsions and also create secondary problems such as worthlessness, trauma to one's sense of self, and in many cases, an identity crisis. As we move toward creating an individualized exposure and response prevention treatment plan, we must be careful not to treat just the obsessions and compulsions. Instead, a successful ERP plan will also address how self-criticism and self-punishment reinforce the O-C cycle, which will, in turn, heal *you*, the whole person.

The Science Behind Self-Criticism

Before you beat yourself up for beating yourself up (yes, this is a common behavior), understand that every human engages in self-criticism, self-blame, and self-punishment. These are also safety behaviors and have been instinctually a part of our survival response for hundreds of thousands of years. When you identify an attribute about yourself that you deem inadequate or unacceptable, your brain will naturally compute this as a major threat to your safety and set off the FFF response. In response to this "inadequacy," you instinctually and automatically respond by criticizing or punishing yourself to self-correct your "badness." This response evolved in early humans because our safety was tied to being accepted as part of our group; we had to avoid being abandoned. Avoiding abandonment has kept us alive. The human species instinctively sees isolation and abandonment as a threat to our survival, so we do whatever we can to avoid it. Similarly, suppose you are disapproved of or criticized by another person. In that case, you might not stop to question the validity of their comment or judgment because, ultimately, their opinion may determine whether you are abandoned or not.

Unfortunately, beyond this survival mechanism, the benefits of self-criticism, self-blame, and self-punishment are minimal. Research has shown that self-criticism increases feelings of inferiority, failure, shame, and guilt and also increases rates of depression, relationship difficulties, low mood, and anxiety disorders (Warren et al. 2016). While these safety behaviors may have originally been performed to correct your flaws and mistakes, you likely became desensitized to this form of motivation quickly. Instead, self-criticism, self-blame, and self-punishment become constant sources of persecution and ridicule and result in many secondary adverse outcomes.

The adverse outcomes of self-criticism, self-blame, and self-punishment are not limited to feeling bad about yourself. Scientific research has shown that these painful behaviors also activate the nervous system's threat detection, signaling your brain to send even more stress hormones throughout your body and resulting in even more anxiety, panic, and hypervigilance (Gilbert 2010). Self-punishment safety behaviors may also involve limiting your self-care and exposure to pleasure, two important practices that can protect you against experiences of shame, guilt, low self-esteem, and depression.

Lastly, we also now have data to show that high levels of self-criticism decrease the outcomes of standard therapies (Rector et al. 2000). This research profoundly confirms my observations as a mental health professional who specializes in treating people with OCD. Those who are hard on themselves are more likely to struggle to engage in exposure and response prevention and are more likely to stop coming to sessions before reaching their treatment goals.

This workbook is written with the goal of helping you, the entire person. Not just your thoughts. Not just your behaviors. But *you* and your relationship with yourself. From this moment on, we (you and I) are on a mission to implement these tools and practices into your life so that you will be able to manage your OCD and also reduce your shame, self-criticism, and self-punishment. This is a journey in which you will develop a better relationship with your anxiety, uncertainty, and doubt, and you will commit to treating yourself with the kindness and respect you have always deserved. This kindness and respect is called *self-compassion.*

What Is Self-Compassion?

Paul Gilbert, one of the pioneering researchers on compassion, defines "compassion" as the "kindness, support, and encouragement that promote the courage we need to take the actions we need in order to promote the flourishing and well-being of ourselves and others." (Gilbert and Choden 2014, p. 98). In simpler terms, self-compassion is simply providing yourself the same sensitivity and unconditional wish of happiness and well-being that you would give a friend or family member for whom you care deeply. The act of self-compassion is emotional, physical, and spiritual.

Alex   "I am confused. I engage in compulsions to relieve my anxiety. If self-compassion is all about relieving our own suffering, why are you asking me to stop my compulsions?"

When we look at the O-C cycle, we can see that compulsions *do* provide relief. This is true. But while compulsions can temporarily relieve your short-term discomfort, uncertainty, and anxiety, they ultimately cause more pain in the long term. Even though they may feel like the kindest thing you can do for yourself when facing extreme anxiety levels, compulsions are not an act of compassion.

Moving Forward

By moving forward, instead of engaging in compulsions and self-criticism, you will learn how to meet and greet the anxiety, uncertainty, and discomfort that you experience with a deep sense of self-respect and self-compassion. By marrying exposure and response prevention with self-compassion, you will have all the tools you need to manage your obsessions and compulsions. Throughout the rest of this workbook, we will call this practice self-compassionate exposure and response prevention (SC-ERP).

Key Points to Remember

- There are key differences in the brain of someone with OCD that make it hard for them to stop intrusive thoughts, images, sensations, feelings, and urges.

- Obsessions are followed by challenging levels of anxiety and uncertainty.

- In an effort to reduce or remove anxiety and uncertainty, people with OCD engage in repetitive safety-seeking compulsions.

- These compulsions do provide short-term relief, but then reinforce the obsession causing long-term discomfort and suffering.

- During this cycle, people with OCD also engage in painful self-criticism and self-punishment, which also reinforces the obsessions and compulsions and causes significant degrees of shame, blame, and feelings of worthlessness.

- The evidence-based way to stop the O-C cycle is to practice facing your fears while practicing the reduction and elimination of compulsions using exposure and response prevention.

- By practicing self-compassion and mindfulness, you can manage your uncertainty and anxiety while also healing the shame, guilt, grief, and sadness that come along with having OCD.

CHAPTER 2

The Core Concepts of Self-Compassion

In the last chapter, you gained an understanding of why you have repetitive and intrusive thoughts, images, feelings, sensations, and urges. You also learned why you often get stuck engaging in safety-seeking compulsions. With this understanding, you can acknowledge that your obsessions do not define who you are as a human and that your compulsive behaviors are instinctive human responses to a glitchy nervous system. With this information, you will move forward, leaving behind the narrative that there was ever something wrong with you, and instead, adopting a deep sense of compassion for yourself. You were put in a confusing situation in which you felt you had no option but to adopt such safety behaviors to avoid what felt like terrorizing danger. None of this is your fault!

With this wisdom, we now move into this chapter acknowledging this truth and committing to breaking this cycle with *fierce self-compassion* and *badassery*.

The First and Second Arrows: A Buddhist Parable

Imagine you are a member of a hunter-gatherer tribe, walking through an open field and gathering berries for your family. All of a sudden, you feel intense pain in your leg. You look down and see that the arrow of a nearby hunter has hit you in the thigh. At one moment, you were experiencing a reasonably normal afternoon gathering berries, and in the next, you are overwhelmed with great pain. This experience is called the "first arrow"—the pain and hardship we experience day in and day out as human beings. These pains are unpredictable and out of our control. As human beings, we will experience many "first arrows" during our lifetime.

After being hit by the "first arrow," we humans often react to our pain by resisting our suffering, judging ourselves critically, or punishing ourselves for being hit by the first arrow. We might say, "You idiot! Look at what you have done. You should have known that this could happen. Why didn't you collect berries elsewhere? Why did you allow this to happen? You are so foolish! Others would have handled this so much better." This reaction is called the "second arrow"—the pain and suffering we cause to ourselves when we react to our suffering with self-judgment, self-criticism, shaming, comparison, and mental rumination. The second arrow is the metaphorical equivalent of stabbing ourselves in the leg, this time with our own arrow.

This Buddhist parable is also a good explanation of the internal process of many with obsessive-compulsive disorder. The first arrows are the intrusive thoughts, feelings, sensations, or urges you automatically experience every day. You will never have control over these first arrows. There is a moment, however, right after you have experienced an intrusive thought, image, feeling, sensation, or urge (first arrow), when you have an opportunity to make some important choices. Do you choose to treat yourself in ways that only create more pain and suffering (second arrow), or do you choose to change the way you respond to your discomfort and meet your suffering (from the first arrow) with kindness, tenderness, and respect? I hope that you will always choose self-compassion.

In this chapter, we will examine the six core concepts of self-compassion that I believe are crucial for your long-term OCD recovery. They are (1) equality, (2) mindfulness, (3) warmheartedness, (4) wisdom, (5) acceptance of imperfection, and (6) compassionate responsibility. Each of these concepts is each equally important and essential in changing the way you treat yourself. While it may feel easier to skip ahead to the concepts that you feel are most relevant to you, I urge you to read through each core concept and consider how it can change the way you see yourself and how you respond to your intrusive thoughts, images, feelings, sensations, and urges.

Equality

Believe it or not, self-compassion is not just about meeting pain with kindness. Self-compassion is a human rights issue and an issue of social equality. You and I—and every other human being—are equal in our worth, and we all are deserving of compassion. The topic of equality is going to be the cornerstone of your self-compassion practice. Let's explore this concept with a story.

When my son was in kindergarten, he and all of his wide-eyed, curious, and vibrant classmates were each given a tall and narrow clip-chart. In the center, a clothespin was attached to the edge of the chart. Above the peg was a series of sections that led to the top section, which said, "Great Job! You made it! ☺" Below the peg was another series of sections leading to the bottom, which said, "Teacher calls your parents. ☹" If you behaved well, your teacher would incrementally "clip up" your clothespin to the next section up. If you "clipped down," your clothespin would move down one section. If you behaved well all day and incrementally moved your peg to the "You made it!" section, you got to have special playtime at the end of the day. Sadly, we all know what happens to the kids whose pin was moved to the bottom section ☹.

The spaces between the ☺, the clothespin, and the ☹ showed different emojis so that the children knew they were either on their way to success or on the way to having an awkward talking to by their parents. My son would often come home proud of himself for being awarded special playtime and would sometimes come home to report that he had come one step away from the "call your mommy" section.

So, you might be wondering what these charts have to do with you and equality? Simply put, when it comes to your worth as a human being, there is no such thing as "clipping up" or "clipping down." Equality means everyone is worthy of love, compassion and respect, no matter what. Equality means that everyone lives at the top, right up there in the "You made it!" section, every single day. Equality means that you are worthy, no matter what thoughts you have, what your mental health status is, no matter what mental or medical diagnosis you have, and no matter your race, sexuality, income, physical ability, social media following, your productivity, or what size body you live in.

While the clip-chart system works really well at managing behavior in a classroom of kindergarteners, it should not be implemented into adulthood as a way of calculating your deservedness for love, compassion, and respect. Unfortunately, our society has collectively adopted this metaphorical clip-chart system and used it to ruin our sense-of-self. Most likely, from a very young age, you also started calculating your worth based on external factors. Using this messy mathematical equation, you lost sight that you are equally deserving of love, compassion, and respect as any other human. Instead, we rank ourselves and each other, telling ourselves that some people rank higher and therefore deserve more than we do and that some rank lower than us, giving us permission to use their situation to make us feel better about ourselves.

The metaphorical clip-chart system mistakenly declares that if you behave in a certain way, not only did you "do good things," but also that you *are* "good." If you perform poorly or fail to meet the standards our society demands of us, this means not only that you did a "bad" thing but also that you *are* "bad." If you have good thoughts, you *are* good, and if you have bad thoughts, you *are* bad. This faulty calculation is where shame is born and thrives, perpetuating a false narrative about who you are, your worth as a human being, and what you deserve.

Equality means that all humans (yes, including you) deserve an abundance of love, kindness, compassion, safety, and respect. I insist that right now you throw out the clip-chart and start treating yourself as an equal. Stop clipping yourself down when you have an intrusive thought or engage in a compulsion. Stop gathering mental lists of all of your "bad" behaviors. Remember, *there is no clip-chart*. Everyone is at the top, and everyone is an equal. Until you throw it out, you will continue to engage in harmful comparison, self-punishment, self-blame, self-criticism, and other hurtful behaviors. Everyone, including you, deserves to be treated with the same degree of respect, compassion, and care. Your worth and deservedness of self-compassion has nothing to do with your mental health status, mental health diagnosis, the thoughts you think, the images you imagine, the sensations you sense, the emotions you feel, the urges you experience, and the compulsions you engage in.

Reflection

Use the space below to reflect on the provided questions about equality.

Using your clip-chart metaphor, in the past, what was required to get to the "Great job! You made it!" section of your clip chart?

_____

_____

_____

_____

Up until this point, what behaviors or events caused you to get "clipped down"?

_____

_____

_____

_____

Can you commit to letting go of the metaphorical clip-chart? What will you need to remind yourself to do so?

_____

_____

_____

_____

Mindfulness

Mindfulness is the act of being present, without judgment. Being mindful means you are aware of your present situation, and you do not attach a story of "good" or "bad" to what you are experiencing. To explain mindfulness in simple terms, let's return to the metaphor of being hit in the leg by the first arrow. As mentioned, being hit by an arrow (your obsessions) is painful and something you never signed up for or have control of. When you experience intrusive thoughts, feelings, sensations, images or urges, you can either resist it and judge them and yourself harshly, causing even more pain (the second arrow), or you can practice being mindful. Being mindful involves several important practices.

One component of being mindful involves first acknowledging that you are in pain. This requires that you become *aware* and in tune with your experience, both physically and emotionally. Becoming aware involves slowing down and recognizing the pain you are in compassionately and tenderly. Once you notice that you are in pain, try not to resist what you are experiencing. Try to remember that the obsessions are not the problem. The problem is resisting and fighting the obsession. Resistance only makes you feel more out of control and more hopeless.

Mindfulness also involves the practice of non-judgment. When you have been hit by the first arrow (your intrusive thoughts, images, sensations, emotions, and urges) and you are in pain (anxious, uncertain, and uncomfortable), judging the pain as "bad," "wrong," or "terrible" will only make the pain and suffering you are experiencing worse. Now, I am not suggesting you go around saying, "I love my obsessions! They are fantastic!" That would not help, as there is nothing fantastic about the obsessions you experience. Instead, practicing non-judgment requires you to acknowledge the obsession and then label it as exactly what it is—an obsession. Just because you are experiencing an obsession does not mean it is bad or dangerous and does not mean you have to do anything about it.

One of the most helpful components of mindfulness when practicing self-compassion and ERP is acknowledging that everything, even the incredibly painful experiences, is temporary. As you practice ERP or your self-compassion skills, you are bound to experience varying degrees of discomfort. Try to be mindful and acknowledge that with time, the discomfort you are feeling will rise and fall on its own. No obsession lasts forever, and your job is to practice allowing your symptoms to come and go as they please, being sure not to push them away.

Being *present* is one of the most essential components of mindfulness. Being present means only attending to this present moment. Not tomorrow. Not two hours from now. Not yesterday. Being present is giving your attention to just *this* moment only. When you have an intrusive thought about something scary happening in the future, instead of following that thought and engaging in things that are not currently happening in this very moment, direct your attention to what *is* happening right now. Let's do an activity to help you with this.

Putting Your Skills into Practice

Using the prompts below, put the mindfulness concepts into action and reflect on your experience. Tanya provided her example responses under each question.

Take a few moments and take a look around. Where are you? What do you see? What shapes do you notice? What colors do you observe?

Tanya: "I am in the office with you. I see your chair. I see the window. I see the silver doorknob. It is an oval shape."

_____

_____

_____

_____

What textures do you notice?

Tanya: "I notice that my jeans feel kind of scratchy, and my skin is soft to touch. I also notice the blanket on the couch is velvety."

_____

_____

_____

_____

Bring your attention to what you hear. What noises do you notice?

Tanya: "I can hear the sound of the cars on the street and the tick-tock of your clock."

_____

_____

_____

_____

Do you notice any distinct smells?

Tanya: "I notice the smell of lavender oil from your diffusor, and I also smell the laundry detergent on my clothes."

_____

_____

_____

_____

What tastes do you taste when you bring your attention to your taste buds?

Tanya: "I notice the taste of toothpaste and a faint taste of coffee from my breakfast."

_____

_____

_____

_____

Connecting with your five senses is one of the best ways to become present. What was it like for you to put your focus on this present moment?

Tanya: "It was nice. It felt like I was awake for my life, just for a few minutes. I have not felt that way in a while. There were a few times when my obsessions started bugging me, but I just brought my attention back to the activities and my senses."

_____

_____

_____

_____

_____

Key Points to Remember

To help remember the core mindfulness tools, Tanya created a "mindfulness cheat sheet" provided below. I understand that these concepts might feel foreign at first, so be gentle with yourself as you learn this new skill. In chapter 3, you will have many opportunities to practice many different mindfulness exercises and meditations to strengthen this skill.

Activating thought, event, or situation	Mindful response
This thought or feeling will never go away.	This thought is temporary and will pass with time.
This thought is "bad."	This thought is neither good nor bad. It is a thought.
I hate this feeling, and I wish it would go away.	This feeling is uncomfortable, and it makes sense I don't enjoy it. However, it is here, so I will practice not fighting it or judging it.
What if my fear comes true and it's all my fault?	I am going to stay present and practice only tending to what is happening right now. I will practice being uncertain and allow myself to feel that uncertainty without judging it as bad or wrong.
But what if this is not OCD?	Again, I am going to stay present. I am going to engage in what I can control and let go of what I cannot control.
I cannot handle this.	I am handling this. I will continue to ride this discomfort out one moment at a time.
I suck at mindfulness and self-compassion.	It is okay that this does not come easily. I will practice non-judgment as I move forward with these practices.

Warmheartedness

Once you are mindful of your suffering, you will respond to the sufferer (you) by connecting to your innate warmheartedness. Warmheartedness is the core practice of self-compassion. Being warmhearted involves meeting you *and* your experience of pain and discomfort with affection, generosity, and sensitivity. You will have many opportunities to connect with your warmheartedness in chapter 3. However, below is an exercise that may give you a glimpse into the compassionate part of you that already exists.

Connecting with the Compassion That Lives Inside You

I want you to bring to mind a dear friend or family member, someone you care deeply about. Now, imagine that they are going through a challenging time with their mental health. Your dear friend is struggling, and they are hard on themselves for what they are going through.

Who is this person you are thinking of?

_____

How does it make you feel to know that they are suffering?

_____

_____

_____

If you could be with them right now, what might you say to them?

_____

_____

_____

What gestures would you make? Would you want to hug them? Put your hand on their hand? Would you smile at them gently? Would you offer to help?

_____

_____

_____

Now, I want you to think back to an instance in the last week when you struggled with a difficult time. How did you treat yourself? What words did you say to yourself?

_____

_____

_____

_____

Did you nurture yourself in the same way you would if your friend was struggling?

_____

_____

_____

You may have found your experience with this exercise to be quite shocking, or maybe you were not surprised at all. Either way, what I hope you learned is that you already know how to access warmheartedness. If you noticed your own inclination to soothe and nurture your friend, even if it was for just a millisecond, you have the capacity for warmheartedness. Warmheartedness lives within you, and with practice, it is a skill you can learn to offer to yourself unconditionally.

If you struggled with this activity and struggled to connect with the warmheartedness that lives inside you, please do not be concerned. Just the intention to connect with your warmheartedness is a fantastic start and is all you need to make your way through this workbook.

If we returned to the first and second arrows story, warmheartedness involves caring for both the wound caused by the first arrow and the emotions that the first arrow created. Warmheartedness would involve saying, "Oh, my dear one, you are in pain. How can I tend to your pain while it rises and falls?" Warmheartedness involves validating the pain you are experiencing and allowing your own love to permeate every part of your being. With each moment of suffering, you will validate the impact it has on you, without blame, criticism, or engaging in behaviors that undermine your experience.

Wisdom

Wisdom is the deep knowledge and understanding of what serves you best in a moment of suffering and pain. When you experience an intrusive thought, image, sensation, urge, or feeling (first arrow), your instincts are going to have you running away from fear, uncertainty, and other perceived dangers as fast as you can. Instead, wisdom would acknowledge that short-term relief from pain will only create more pain later (second arrow), and instead, wisdom would have you lean into that fear. Wisdom involves reflection and learning from past experiences. It is the act of recognizing what serves you well emotionally, physically, and spiritually. Wisdom asks the question, "What is it that you need during this difficult time?" and is willing to listen, even if the answer is not what you want to hear.

I believe that everyone, even youngsters, can develop deep wisdom for their well-being. Through trial and error, we can learn what works and what does not work. In fact, that is why making mistakes or noticing our erroneous patterns are awesome! Wisdom involves seeing trends in behaviors that are not working and then having the willingness to take the hard road, not as a form of self-punishment, but as a sign of respect for what will bring you a long-term reduction of pain and suffering.

Wisdom also involves identifying exactly *why* you are choosing your behaviors. When you begin to engage in ERP, you will need to be clear on why you are choosing to lean into your fear, as this will help motivate you and keep you on track.

Todd   Todd had been engaging in exposure and response prevention for a few weeks and came to my office quite confused and angry. He reported, "I just don't understand how it benefits me to purposely face my anxiety and uncertainty when I am already in so much distress! This week, all I could think was, *Why am I doing this to myself?* I was so worked up last night. I wanted to punch something."

I had so much empathy and compassion for Todd. He was doing really hard work in therapy while also trying to keep up his grades and not miss basketball practices. I used this as a perfect opportunity for Todd to connect with his inner wisdom. I asked him a few questions hoping that his own wisdom would guide him through his suffering without my jumping in and rescuing him from his distress. I responded by saying, "Todd, I can see that you are being met with a profound degree of pain right now while also trying to keep up with your ERP and your daily functioning. It really is quite remarkable. I wonder if you could reflect on this situation, and you tell me *why* you are engaging in exposure and response prevention at this time?" It didn't take long for Todd to identify the many things OCD had taken from him. Todd also reflected and recognized that the impact OCD had on his life far outweighed the challenges of ERP.

Reflection

In the space on the next page, reflect on the prompts provided.

How has OCD impacted your life? How has it impacted your relationships, career, academics, hobbies, quality of life, self-esteem, and so on?

A few of Todd's responses:

"OCD has

- stopped me from seeing my friends,

- taken the joy out of the things I love to do,

- interrupted my studies, causing my grades to drop,

- caused me to hate myself, and

- impacted my parents' lives and well-being."

_____

_____

_____

_____

Using these points, write a powerful statement declaring *why* you are committed to staring your fears in the face and willingly engaging in self-compassionate ERP.

Todd: "I refuse to let OCD take my life away from me. I will do the exact opposite of what OCD wants me to do, because running away from fear only makes me feel awful and moves me further from the things I love to do. I am going to practice being kind to myself because that is what I deserve and that is the wise thing to do."

_____

_____

_____

_____

Knowing your *why* is a crucial aspect of self-compassion, as self-compassion involves leaning into pain and not escaping it. Wisdom is knowing when to lean in and why you are choosing to do so.

Imperfection

As humans, demanding that we be perfect or get an A+ at everything usually creates suffering. In many cases, it causes severe, debilitating pain and distress. While it is true that you can achieve a perfect score on a test or sometimes experience a "perfect" moment, expecting yourself to be perfect frequently ends in painful disappointment. Either you don't reach the perfect goal, or—even if you *do* reach it—you will still likely have continued anxiety, because you have to maintain this perfect behavior in the future.

Instead of always aiming for an A+, give yourself permission to aim for a more compassionate B-. Yes, you read that correctly! In life, I strongly encourage you to aim for no higher than a B-. There are no exceptions to this rule, and believe it or not, I am even going to encourage you to try to get a B- in your self-compassion practices. Endlessly aiming for an A+ will only set you up to be critical of yourself and continuously dissatisfied and disappointed.

Allow things to get a little messy. Give yourself permission to be less than perfect for a change. Offer yourself self-compassion for your imperfections and give yourself some time to rest and just be. Instead of expecting only "good" thoughts or feelings, settle for having a whole range of thoughts and emotions. Let go of trying to get people's approval, and give yourself permission to be just who you are, a human being who makes mistakes, but whose heart is genuine and enough. Setting realistic expectations is one of the most compassionate things we can do for ourselves. Life gets a whole lot better when you drop the A+ mentality and aim for a B-.

Todd   "Taking a B- mentality is the most ridiculous idea I have ever heard in my lifetime. How do you expect me to get into a good college and succeed with a B- mentality?"

Todd raises an important point. What do you do if you need to give a presentation at work or take an important test? These outcomes matter, right? Yes, this is true. It is first important to address the pros and cons of Todd's perfectionism. Was it helping more than it was hindering? Were the benefits of pushing himself to the absolute maximum worth it in the long term? After some consideration, Todd agreed that his perfectionism was not only making his OCD worse but also interfering with his friendships and quality of life. Todd reported he was not even able to get through his homework without having a panic attack.

Todd and I looked at ways he could motivate himself other than forcing an A+ mentality. Todd discovered that he could still perform at outstandingly high levels without setting unhealthy, perfectionistic expectations or engaging in harmful negative self-talk. When Todd had anxiety-producing thoughts about exams or basketball games (first arrows), he pivoted away from engaging in compulsive re-reading of school materials or compulsively practicing layups and free throws. Instead, Todd used his wisdom to determine what actions are effective and what are not. Once he had made a wise choice, he chose to meet his anticipatory anxiety with warmheartedness.

Reflection

What areas of your life do you expect perfection?

_____

_____

Do these expectations improve or harm your emotional well-being?

_____

_____

_____

What are you afraid will happen if you embrace a B- mindset?

_____

_____

_____

Are there any areas of your life where you are willing to embrace a B-? If so, what would change?

_____

_____

_____

Compassionate Responsibility

If we return to the definition of "self-compassion," you may recall that self-compassion involves the deep wish to take care of yourself and relieve your suffering. I am sure you can agree; having a deep wish to alleviate your suffering is easy. This desire to live a better life is most likely what prompted you to pick up this workbook. The hard part is executing the plan. For this reason, the final core concept of self-compassion is called "compassionate responsibility."

Compassionate responsibility is the act of genuinely putting yourself first for the sake of your well-being and quality of life. Taking compassionate responsibility is putting you as the number-one priority and being the first person to offer yourself compassion in a time of need. You are doing this not because no one cares about you but because you want to create a relationship with yourself in which you will have your own back—any time, anywhere. Taking compassionate responsibility is being unconditionally there for yourself, even when you are exhausted and have nothing left to give. It's bold. It's unconditional. And it's badass!

Tanya   Tanya was having a challenging time with her OCD, and her partner, Julie, wanted nothing more than to take Tanya's pain away. Tanya shared that she found great comfort in reaching out to Julie when she was anxious. Asking Julie to support her made her feel loved. Tanya and I marveled at how nice it was that she had a partner who cared for her so much, but I asked her, "I wonder if there is a chance you could be the first person to soothe and tend to your struggles before seeking out Julie for support?" Tanya looked confused. "Why would I try to support myself when Julie does it so much better than I? I feel so much stronger after she sits with me and hugs me." I validated Tanya and agreed that there is nothing better than being loved and supported by another person. However, I asked Tanya to consider if that helps her in the long term. Could Tanya own that her anxiety is hers, and instead of criticizing herself or going to her partner, could she take the ultimate act of being her own number-one support system?

This was life changing for Tanya, and it could be for you too. Taking compassionate responsibility involves taking 100 percent responsibility for your recovery, again, not because you don't deserve a loved one's warmth and tenderness, but because you deserve *your* warmth and tenderness. Your long-term recovery is going to be largely based on how much you put this core concept into practice by responding compassionately to your suffering. So I pose the same question to you: "Can you commit to always being the first person to soothe and tend to your struggles?"

Being Your Own Kind Coach

As you proceed into the rest of this workbook, you are going to engage in dozens of self-compassion and ERP practices. To do this, you will need to motivate yourself, as these practices are challenging and require a certain degree of accountability and self-coaching. When I talk about coaching, I am not talking about some kind of drill sergeant who yells at you and puts you down. We all know how that feels. Awful! To get you through the tough times and the high levels of anxiety and uncertainty, I will ask you to employ what I like to call your "kind coach." Your kind coach does not yell. They use their stellar coaching skills to encourage you, cheer for you, and remind you why you are here, doing this really hard work. Your kind coach knows what your strengths are and champions you by reminding you of each and every one of them. Your kind coach also knows your weaknesses and knows not to use them against you during challenging times. They are committed to your long-term recovery and genuinely want what is best for you.

During the next chapter, and throughout the rest of this workbook, you will have many opportunities to practice accessing the qualities of your kind coach and practicing the other five core self-compassion concepts. You might find that you are already employing some of these core concepts, or you might find that you need to practice all of them. Using the space below, journal down your reflections to the provided questions

Chapter Reflection

Which core concept do you feel you need to practice the most?

_____

_____

What can you do to support your growth in this area? How might you remind yourself of this core concept?

_____

_____

_____

_____

Is there a core concept that did not sit well with you? If so, why?

_____

_____

CHAPTER 3

Daily Self-Compassion Practices

Deep inside you lives a compassionate presence that is wise, warm, and unconditional. This compassionate presence, your compassionate self, has always been inside you. At some point in your life, your compassionate self started having to compete with societal and cultural messages that made you question the wisdom of your compassionate self and expect ideals such as success, popularity, and perfection—a perfect body and perfect thoughts, behaviors, and mental health (Remember the clip-chart?). In addition, the volume of your intrusive, repetitive thoughts became so loud that, over time, your nurturing, soothing, compassionate self was quieted.

Reconnecting to your compassionate self will require you to listen very carefully. Its voice is likely to be faint at first, causing you to question if it is even there. You will need to remind yourself that your compassionate self always has and always will be there for you, ready to support and care for you in times of need. As you work toward befriending your compassionate self again, please remember that your goal should not be to make your obsessions or societal messages disappear. That would only end in a tug-of-war with your thoughts and feelings. Instead, this work is about identifying when you are suffering and calling upon the compassionate wisdom that lives inside you. Don't give up!

How to Use This Chapter

This chapter is broken into two sections: self-compassion practices and self-compassion meditations. These exercises are organized with the goal of your being able to easily access self-compassion in your daily life and reconnecting with the compassionate self that exists inside you. I encourage you to experiment with each exercise and incorporate as many as possible into your daily routine. If a particular practice or meditation does not resonate with you, it is entirely okay to move on to another exercise. When you are ready, come back to it and reflect on what it is about the practice you did not like. Sometimes the exercises we struggle with are the ones that teach us the most. In this chapter, Simone will walk alongside you and give you some examples of her own self-compassion practices.

As you go through the practices in this chapter, please be patient with yourself. This process is like growing a garden. The seeds of compassion are already there, ready to be tended to and nurtured. Once watered, these seeds will need time to germinate under the soil's surface before they can make their way up to the light. If you don't see any progress right away, this could be because your self-compassion is cultivating a strong root system before it is ready to show you its true nature. Don't give up! Your compassionate self is there, and its voice will return with time.

Self-Compassion Practices for Fear, Uncertainty, and Doubt

Visualizing Your Compassionate Self

Visualizing your compassionate self—cultivating a compassionate image—is a foundational practice of compassion-focused therapy (Gilbert and Choden 2014). This practice aims at identifying an image of unconditional affection and softheartedness that can be accessed during any time of need. Paul Gilbert, the founder of compassion-focused therapy, states that when you use an image of your compassionate self and are "in its presence, you can be yourself; there is no need to pretend to be what you are not. It completely understands you, accepts you, and is loving toward you" (Gilbert and Choden 2014, 243).

Putting Your Skills into Practice

Take a moment to settle in, gently giving your attention to your breath. See if you can find a rhythm with your breathing or notice the rise and fall of your chest as you breathe.

Remind yourself that you deserve to be here and that you deserve to provide yourself with kindness and a loving presence.

While you allow your thoughts, feelings, sensations, and urges to come and go as they please, imagine being filled with a sense of warmth, kindness, and protection and ponder on the below questions.

Using the space below, journal your reflections on the questions provided.

Does your compassionate self have a masculine or feminine voice? Or another voice? What is the tone of your compassionate self—soft, deep, loud, sweet, tender, or something else? If you are struggling to identify the answers to these prompts, simply write what you wish it sounded like. Again, just the intention of connecting with your compassionate self is enough.

Simone: "My compassionate self has a soft, feminine voice. In fact, it is my voice, but also sounds a little like my grandmother. My compassionate self is wise."

_____

_____

_____

How would you like your compassionate self to relate to you?

Simone: "My compassionate self wants what is best for me and believes in me. My compassionate self stands up for me when I am struggling."

_____

_____

_____

How would you like to relate to your compassionate self?

Simone: "I would like to trust my compassionate self. I would like to listen to it instead of listening to OCD and the harsh things I say to myself."

_____

_____

_____

How can your compassionate self show you its commitment to your emotional wellness?

Simone: "My compassionate self protects me and fights for me and my wellness. It is like a momma bear and a papa bear all tied into one."

_____

_____

_____

What do you genuinely need to feel a deep sense of tenderness and safety from your compassionate self?

Simone: "I need to embrace that I am worthy and lovable, even when I have thoughts that disgust me."

_____

_____

_____

If you openly shared everything you are going through with your compassionate friend, what would you like them to say to you? Try not to hold back your genuine answer because of the potential awkwardness or vulnerability you might feel. Give yourself permission to reveal what you really need to hear.

Simone: "I would like my compassionate self to sit with me while I cried and grieved all that I have lost from OCD. I would like it to validate me and how scary this is for me. I would like my compassionate self to tell me how strong I am and that it will never leave my side."

_____

_____

_____

The Language of Compassion

Many find that the practice of self-compassion brings with it an entirely new language. Instead of using words like "should" and "can't" and other words that promote self-blame and self-criticism, you will now practice using words of kindness, warmth, and unconditional care. Many who embark on this practice find that they have a limited self-compassion vocabulary.

Putting Your Skills into Practice

Below is a list of words that may help you connect with your compassionate self. You will find some words to be soothing while others might make you slightly uncomfortable. Experiment with saying each word aloud or silently to yourself. Circle the words that you would like to add to your daily vocabulary.

Affectionate	Goodness	Sincere
Caress	Heart-centered	Softheartedness
Considerate	Kind	Sweetheart
Darling	Loving	Sweetness
Dear one	Loving-kindness	Tenderheartedness
Delicate	Mellifluous	Tenderness
Empathic	Nurture	Thoughtfulness
Fondness	Open	Unconditional love
Gentle	Openness	Warmth
Genuine	Peacefulness	

When you have anxiety, you might notice that it is difficult to access self-compassion because you are flooded by your biological fight-flight-or-freeze response. Your threat system is preparing you to defend yourself from the perceived threat. A simple practice that can bring you back to a nurturing and compassionate state of mind is to simply ask yourself, "What would my compassionate self say to me right now?" If this is difficult, you may simply ask, "What would I like to hear a loved one whisper in my ear at this time?"

Simone's Compassionate Reframe Statements

- I am not alone.

- It is okay that you are scared right now. I am here for you.

- I am noticing that anxiety and uncertainty just arose. I have what it takes to ride this anxiety out.

- I love you. I am here for you while this fear rises and falls on its own.

- I deserve unconditional warmth and kindness, no matter what thoughts I have.

- May I offer myself support during this difficult moment.

- This is not easy for me. May I offer myself love at this time.

- May I be kind to myself while this feeling accompanies me throughout this day.

- I am here for you, no matter how hard things get.

- I will not leave your side. I have your back always.

- May I be open to receiving self-compassion (this is often helpful for those who cannot find an answer to the question or access compassion at this time).

Reflection

In the space below, write a few statements that you think you would like to hear in the future when you are facing fear, uncertainty, and doubt.

_____

_____

_____

_____

_____

_____

Next time you are met with anxiety, uncertainty, or fear, ask yourself, "What would my compassionate self say to me right now?" and see if you can access a moment of tenderness toward yourself. If you like, you may also say your compassionate reframe aloud and see if that lands deeper within you. You can even rehearse your compassionate reframe so you can become more familiar with what your compassionate self would say in different situations.

Taking a Self-Compassion Break

One of my favorite self-compassion practices is taking a self-compassion break. This practice, developed by Kristin Neff and Christopher Germer (2018), reminds us to use the three components of their mindful self-compassion practices: mindfulness, common humanity, and self-kindness. The following exercise comes from Neff and Germer's *Mindful Self-Compassion Workbook*, and is used with permission.

Putting Your Skills into Practice

Think of a situation in your life that is causing you stress, such as a health problem, relationship problem, work problem, or some other struggle. Choose a problem in the mild to moderate range, not a big problem, as we want to build the resource of self-compassion gradually.

Visualize the situation clearly in your mind's eye. What is the setting? Who is saying what to whom? What is happening? What might happen? Can you feel discomfort in your body as you bring this difficulty to mind? If not, choose a slightly more difficult problem.

Now, try saying to yourself: *This is a moment of suffering*. That's mindfulness. Perhaps other wording speaks to you better. Some options are: *This hurts. Ouch. This is stressful*.

Now, try saying to yourself: *Suffering is a part of life*. That's common humanity. Other options include: *I'm not alone. Everyone experiences this, just like me. This is how it feels when people struggle in this way.*

Now, offer yourself the gesture of soothing touch that you discovered in the previous exercise.

And try saying to yourself: *May I be kind to myself* or *May I give myself what I need*. Perhaps there are particular words of kindness and support that you need to hear right now in this difficult situation.

Some options may be:

May I accept myself as I am.

May I begin to accept myself as I am.

May I forgive myself.

May I be strong.

May I be patient.

If you're having difficulty finding the right words, imagine that a dear friend or loved one is having the same problem as you. What would you say to this person? What simple message would you like to deliver to your friend, heart to heart?

Now see if you can offer the same message to yourself.

Simone's Self-Compassion Break Statement:

- "I am feeling anxiety right now (mindfulness). It's okay that I feel this way. All humans experience anxiety. I am not alone (common humanity). May I be gentle with myself as I experience this (self-kindness)."

- "This is a moment of suffering (mindfulness). Suffering is a part of life. I am not alone (common humanity). I will offer myself compassion and will try not to judge myself harshly (self-kindness)."

- "I feel sad and angry that I have OCD (mindfulness). I am sure everyone with OCD often feels this way at times (common humanity). May I be gentle with myself and honor how hard this is (self-kindness)."

Reflection

In the space below, write your complete self-compassion break statement.

_____

_____

_____

_____

_____

_____

_____

Many find it helpful to write their self-compassion break statement in the notes on their phone (or on paper) and read it (aloud or quietly) as often as their heart desires. You could also write your statement on a sticky note and put it in your wallet or post it on your bathroom mirror or anywhere you may need to hear it. One more idea is to create an image with your self-compassion break statement and upload it as the screen saver on your computer or phone. Lastly, it can be really healing to record yourself slowly and tenderly reading your statement and listen back to it when you need to connect with your compassionate self. These are all ideas that you can use with any activity and might deepen your self-compassion practice.

Nurturing Your Suffering with Physical Touch

We know, scientifically, that our nervous system can be soothed through the act of physical touch (Neff 2012). This can be particularly helpful when you find yourself in a painful situation, and you have already engaged in critical self-talk or self-punishment. Compassionate physical touch can be a great way to access your compassionate self without using words or phrases. Instead, it is simply tending to your needs by giving and receiving your own tender physical contact.

Putting Your Skills into Practice

Gently bring your attention to your body and experiment with these different acts of self-compassion through touch:

- Raise the palm of your hand flat on your chest and offer your heart a gentle touch. Hold it to your heart when you need to connect to your compassionate self.

- Using the tips of your fingers, experiment with touching different areas of your body (examples below). Take as much time as you need for this exercise, as it can be so incredibly healing.

  - Hold your cheeks gently with your palms.

  - Run your fingers over your forearm, up to your shoulders.

  - Gently apply pressure to different parts of your feet, ankles, or legs.

  - Run your fingers over your forehead, down over your nose, and down to your lips.

- If there is an area of your body you do not feel comfortable touching, that is entirely okay. Just offer yourself this opportunity to access self-compassion through soothing touch.

- Try using different gestures of self-compassion such as hugging yourself, holding your head with your hands.

- As you touch different areas of your body, try softening any tension you are holding in your body.

Reflection

In the space below, reflect on your experience with compassionate touch. What felt nurturing? What did not?

_____

_____

_____

_____

_____

_____

_____

Things to Consider

If you experience sensorimotor obsessions that are hyper-focused on specific sensations in the body, you may find these practices difficult. This is also the case for those who experience pedophilia or sexual obsessions where the obsessions are hyper-focused on particular parts of the body, such as one's genitals or other erogenous zones. Please give yourself permission to skip these practices if you are not yet ready to practice these skills right now. You will find that these skills will serve you greatly later on, in exposures. When you are ready to begin exposure and response prevention, return to these practices and use them as an opportunity to tolerate the feared sensations while engaging in compassionate physical touch.

Also, these body-focused practices might be difficult if you have a co-occurring disorder such as body dysmorphic disorder, trichotillomania, excoriation disorder, or an eating disorder. Feel free to move on to another practice or consult with a trained mental health professional if you need more support in these areas.

Writing Letters from Your Compassionate Self

Compassionate letter writing is a beautiful practice that will help you develop a deep awareness of how you would like your compassionate self to communicate with you in difficult times. With compassionate letter writing, you will identify and validate your struggles and then express your unconditional self-compassion using a language that feels right to you. Below are some prompts to help you write your letter:

- Your letter might first show an awareness of the struggle you are having.

- Then, add words of unconditional love and kindness.

- You might also show empathy for the distress you are in and acknowledge that you are not alone in this experience.

- Explore helpful solutions that can help you cope. Try to suggest constructive ideas that implement self-compassion.

- As you write this letter (and later read it), remind yourself that this letter is a reflection of you at your wisest and most mature.

- The words you use will be caring, thoughtful, and unconditional.

- As you write, try to soften your face, embracing yourself as a warm and gentle person.

- Try to use words that are warm and encouraging and that resonate with you.

- Your writing does not need to be perfect.

- Compassionate letter writing is all about intention to access your compassionate self. If your intention is there, that is all that matters.

Putting Your Skills into Practice

First, identify an event in the last week where you were particularly hard on yourself.

_____

Using your compassionate self to guide you, write a compassionate letter to yourself in the space below.

Simone:

> Dear Me,
>
> I know my intrusive thoughts are relentless and make me feel anxious, uncertain, and down on myself. Remember, no matter what thoughts I have, I will be right here supporting myself. I deserve warmth and peace of mind. It makes total sense that I have had such a hard time with these thoughts. My brain is simply trying to protect me. Sometimes it gets all worked up and makes things feel extremely dangerous. Many others have OCD and feel similar to me.
>
> I promise to be kind and gentle as I practice allowing this anxiety to be here. I have everything I need to get through this. It is my responsibility to manage my OCD. I know I can tolerate this discomfort, especially if I am self-compassionate.
>
> With warmth and everlasting care,
>
> Me.

Dear _____,

_____

_____

_____

_____

_____

_____

_____

_____

_____

_____

_____

Once your letter is written, read it aloud to yourself in your warmest voice. Using the format given, or one of your own, try to practice compassionate letter writing every day. You may want to write a letter for past events, current events, or future events you are anticipating.

RAIN: A Helpful Self-Compassion Acronym

Tara Brach, an author and meditation teacher, adapted the mindfulness acronym RAIN (for *Recognize, Allow, Investigate, Nurture*) to include the practice of self-compassion. In her book *Radical Compassion*, Brach explains that "the first two steps of RAIN, Recognize and Allow, are the foundation of mindful awareness and compassion. The second two steps, Investigate and Nurture, deepen mindfulness and directly activate compassion" (2019).

Putting Your Skills into Practice

RAIN gives us a step-by-step process of wading through anxiety, uncertainty, and other strong emotions using the practice of mindfulness and self-compassion.

The first step of RAIN—*recognize*—is to recognize what is going on in this present moment, nonjudgmentally. What do you feel? What are you doing? What thoughts are you having? How are you responding to those thoughts? Many of us rush through the day without checking in and recognizing the way things really are. Right now, what are you recognizing?

_____

_____

_____

This second step—*allow*—encourages you to allow whatever is happening in this present moment. If you have intrusive thoughts or sensations that bother you, try to allow them to come and go as they please. Allowing is not just something you say to yourself. Allowing involves a heartfelt intention to let the emotion be in your presence. Remember, just because it is unpleasant does not mean it does not belong. Take a few moments (or as long as you can) to gently allow whatever it is that you are experiencing. What got in the way?

_____

_____

_____

This third step in RAIN—*investigate*—is to examine the thoughts, feelings, sensations, and urges that are in this present moment. This investigation is to spark your *curiosity*, not your analytical mind. Go back to the basics and investigate what you are experiencing as if it were the first time you've ever experienced it. In Zen Buddhist teachings, this curiosity is called "beginner's mind." The beginner's mind involves being open and nonjudgmental, dropping preconceived ideas and beliefs about what you are experiencing. Examples of investigating might be, "How interesting! When I allow my anxiety to be here, it does seem to get worse for a little, but then it starts to fade" or "I am noticing that I *really* tighten my jaw muscles when I feel anxiety rise in my body." Take a few minutes to practice investigating this present moment with curiosity. What did you observe?

_____

_____

_____

This final step of RAIN—*nurture*—encourages you to comfort yourself in this present moment. As humans, when we are met with suffering, we resist it. When we practice *nurturing* ourselves, we meet our suffering with love and tenderheartedness. Take some time (as long as you need) to practice nurturing the suffering you are currently experiencing. Did you notice a shift when you nurtured yourself instead of resisting it?

_____

_____

_____

Brach also explains, "after the RAIN, we shift from the doing to being." This statement explains the importance of not going back to hurrying yourself away from your suffering. In the moments following RAIN, your job is to stay tender and to nurture your discomfort with loving presence, despite how repetitive and painful the thoughts, emotions, and sensations are.

Self-Compassionate Meditations

In the second half of this chapter, I'll lead you through six self-compassionate meditations. You may access the audio recordings of me reading many of these meditations on the website for this book (http://www.newharbinger.com/47766), but I also strongly encourage you to take some time to record yourself reading the provided meditation scripts. More often than not, hearing these words of kindness in your own voice can be the voice you need to hear most.

As you practice these meditations, your intrusive thoughts, images, feelings, sensations, and urges will likely pop in and try and take over. Try to consider your obsessions like clouds in the sky, floating by at their own pace. There is nothing you need to do about them. Your thoughts, images, feelings, sensations, and urges are not important and do not disqualify you from meeting your pain with self-compassion. The more your obsessions come, the more you lean in and tend to your discomfort with self-compassion.

Simone   Simone was finding the self-compassion skills to be helpful so far. However, sometimes during meditation, Simone experienced a spike in her anxiety. Simone would start to panic and ask if we could stop the exercise. Simone was frustrated and shared, "Something is wrong with me. Meditation feels like it is making it worse."

This experience is commonly known as "relaxation-induced anxiety" and is not an indicator that something is wrong. Some people with anxiety can be sensitive to spikes in emotion, especially when moving from an anxious state to a more relaxed state. This does not mean you should give up—quite the opposite, actually. Continued exposure to meditation and relaxation exercises often results in habituation to this contrasting sensitivity and, in turn, a better relationship with anxiety and other difficult emotions.

Things to Consider

- Be aware that meditation practices can sometimes become compulsive. In this case, meditation is used to neutralize or suppress intrusive, violent, or taboo thoughts. If you find that this practice—or any practice in this book, for that matter—becomes a form of thought suppression, reassurance, or a neutralizing compulsion, take a break and come back at a later time when you can willingly tolerate your obsessions.

- People with sensorimotor obsessions often experience hyperawareness of particular sensations in their body—the breath being the most common symptom. Some meditation practices can cause an increased hyperawareness, leading to mental rumination about when one should breathe and what is considered "the right kind of breathing." If this is the case for you, I invite you to use these exercises gently. The practice of meditation might be considered one of the most difficult exposures for you at this time. Aim at slowly introducing these practices and work your way up to being able to engage entirely, just like you would with any other exposure.

Compassionate Friend Meditation

The compassionate friend meditation is an excellent practice for those who are having a hard time accessing self-compassion. Created by Neff and Germer (2018), the compassionate friend meditation focuses on visualizing being cared for by a kind, compassionate friend. You may find this visualization meditation easy or difficult. There is no "right" way to feel or experience this meditation, and it is okay if you struggle to envision your compassionate friend. Even if you have one fleeting image of your compassionate friend flash through your mind, consider that progress! The following exercise comes from Neff and Germer's *Mindful Self-Compassion Workbook* (2018), and is used with permission.

Putting Your Skills into Practice

Find a comfortable position, either sitting or lying down. Gently close your eyes. Take a few deep breaths to settle into your body. Put one or two hands over your heart or another soothing place to remind yourself to give yourself loving attention.

Safe Place

Imagine yourself in a place that is safe and comfortable—it might be a cozy room with the fireplace burning or a peaceful beach with warm sun and a cool breeze, or a forest glade. It could also be an imaginary place, like floating on clouds…anywhere you feel peaceful and safe. Let yourself linger with and enjoy the feeling of comfort in this place.

Compassionate Friend

Soon you'll receive a visitor, a warm and caring presence—a compassionate friend—an imaginary figure who embodies the qualities of wisdom, strength, and unconditional love.

This being may be a spiritual figure or a wise, compassionate teacher; she may embody qualities of someone you have known in the past, like a loving grandparent, or be completely from your imagination. This being may not have any particular form, perhaps just a presence or glowing light.

Your compassionate friend cares deeply about you and would like you to be happy and free from unnecessary struggle.

Allow an image to come to mind.

Arrival

You have a choice to go out from your safe place and meet your compassionate friend or to invite him in. Take that opportunity now, if you like.

Position yourself in just the right way in relation to your compassionate friend—whatever feels right. Then allow yourself to feel what it's like to be in the company of this being. There is nothing you need to do except to experience the moment.

See if you can allow yourself to fully receive the unconditional love and compassion this being has for you, to soak it in. If you can't let it fully in, that's okay too—this being feels it anyway.

Meeting

Your compassionate friend is wise and all-knowing and understands exactly where you are in your own life journey. Your friend might want to tell you something, something that is just what you need to hear right now. Take a moment and listen carefully to what your compassionate friend has come to say. If no words come, that's okay, too—just experience the good company. That's a blessing in itself.

And perhaps you would like to say something to your compassionate friend. Your friend will listen deeply and completely understands you. Is there anything you'd like to share?

Your friend may also like to leave you with a gift—a material object. The object will simply appear in your hands, or you can put out your hands and receive one—something that has special meaning to you. If something appears, what is it?

Now take a few more moments to enjoy your friend's presence. And as you continue to enjoy this being's good company, allow yourself to realize that your friend is actually part of yourself. All the compassionate feelings, images, and words that you experienced flow from your own inner wisdom and compassion.

Return

Finally, when you're ready, allow the images to gradually dissolve in your mind's eye, remembering that compassion and wisdom are always within you, especially when you need them the most. You can call on your compassionate friend anytime you wish.

Now settle back into your body, letting yourself savor what just happened, perhaps reflecting on the words you may have heard or the object that may have been given to you.

And finally, let go of the meditation and allow yourself to feel whatever you feel and to be exactly as you are.

Gently open your eyes.

Reflection

In the space below, write any details you visualized about your compassionate friend.

Who was it? What did they say?

_____

_____

What did you say to your compassionate friend?

_____

_____

_____

_____

_____

What were some of the qualities of your compassionate friend?

_____

_____

What gets in the way of you accessing your compassionate friend? Did you notice any resistance?

_____

_____

Loving-Kindness Meditation

Loving-kindness meditations are widely considered to be one of the most important meditations for developing compassion. Loving-kindness meditations strengthen one's capacity for tenderness, forgiveness, and connection toward ourselves and others.

Putting Your Skills into Practice

Gently bring your attention to your breath or another object that grounds you. If possible, allow yourself to soften any areas where you feel tension. You may also offer yourself a loving touch at this time. And now, slowly, gently, and affectionately offer yourself these phrases.

May I be filled with loving-kindness.

May I be safe from inner and outer dangers.

May I be well in body and mind.

May I be at ease and happy.

As you practice these phrases, imagine your heart radiating loving-kindness to your entire body. You may also offer yourself your own personal loving-kindness phrase. As you practice this meditation, note any word, posture, or gesture that permeates kindness throughout your body and mind.

It is entirely okay if this meditation feels awkward or forced. You may also notice emotions that don't feel anything like loving-kindness. As each emotion arises, offer it loving-kindness. If you notice that obsessions are interfering with this practice, that is okay also. Gently note the presence of the thought, image, feeling, sensation, or urge and offer it the below statements.

May I give myself permission to fully allow this experience.

May I offer myself unconditional kindness at this moment.

May I offer myself warmth and tenderness as I work on my OCD.

Once again, try not to judge yourself during this process. If you would like, widen your offering of loving-kindness to include others. You may send loving-kindness to someone you love, to those who have OCD, or to all living beings. Offer them all the below phrases:

May we be filled with loving-kindness.

May we be safe from inner and outer dangers.

May we be well in body and mind.

May we be at ease and happy.

As you near the end of this meditation, gently offer yourself permission to be imperfect in these self-compassion practices and our lives.

Simone   After practicing this meditation at home, Simone reported the urge to use the phrase "May I be safe from inner and outer dangers" as a compulsion. Simone found herself beginning to repeat this phrase to try to remove her anxiety and uncertainty.

Remember, OCD can be sneaky. If you notice that some of these phrases (or meditations) are being done in an attempt to reduce or remove anxiety, uncertainty, or other form of discomfort, slow down and see if you can bring your attention back to simply meeting each thought, image, feeling, sensation or urge with compassion. This act of compassion should be an attempt to lean into your discomfort and uncertainty, not lean away from it.

Affectionate Breathing

Our breath is something we take with us everywhere. With practice and patience, your breath can become your most reliable friend. In moments of anxiety and uncertainty, your breath can be your anchor and your compass simultaneously. Affectionate breathing, a meditation developed by Neff and Germer (2018), is a meditation that couples bringing attention to the breath with affectionate awareness. The following exercise comes from Neff and Germer's *Mindful Self-Compassion Workbook* (2018), and is used with permission.

Putting Your Skills into Practice

Find a posture in which your body is comfortable and will feel supported for the length of the meditation. Then let your eyes gently close, partially or fully. Take a few slow, easy breaths, releasing any unnecessary tension in your body.

If you like, try placing a hand over your heart or another soothing place as a reminder that we're bringing not only awareness, but affectionate awareness, to our breathing and to ourselves. You can leave your hand there or put it back down at any time.

Begin to notice your breathing in your body, feeling your body breathe in and feeling your body breathe out.

Notice how your body is nourished on the inbreath and relaxes with the outbreath.

See if you can just let your body breathe you. There is nothing you need to do.

Now start to notice the rhythm of your breathing, flowing in and flowing out. Take some time to feel the natural rhythm of your breathing.

Feel your whole body subtly moving with the breath, like the movement of the sea.

Your mind will naturally wander like a curious child or a little puppy. When that happens, just gently return to the rhythm of your breathing.

Allow your whole body to be gently rocked and caressed—internally caressed—by your breathing.

If it feels right, you can give yourself over to your breathing, letting your breathing be all there is. Just breathing. Being breathing.

And now, gently release your attention on your breath, sitting quietly in your own experience, and allow yourself to feel whatever you're feeling and to be just as you are.

Slowly and gently open your eyes.

Compassionate Body Scan

The compassionate body scan can be a beneficial meditation when dealing with high levels of anxiety and uncertainty. This exercise aims to make space for the discomfort in your body and gently meet that discomfort with a deep sense of compassion and positive regard.

Putting Your Skills into Practice

Find a position that feels comfortable for you. Slowly bring your attention to your breath and begin to notice how your breath allows your chest to rise and fall.

Gently close your eyes and imagine that your body is made of beautiful, transparent tempered glass. The glass forms the shape of your body, creating a silhouette, similar to a body-shaped vase. Now, imagine that your glass body is being filled with the clearest, warmest water.

Now, I want you to imagine a tiny hole, maybe the size of a pinhole, on the bottom of both of your big toes. Using this image, visualize that this warm water is draining slowly out of your big toes.

Slowly bring your attention to the top of your head and imagine the level of the warm water getting lower and moving past your forehead as it slowly drains out of your body. As the warmth of the water slowly moves past your forehead, send warmth and appreciation to that area of your body. If uncomfortable thoughts and feelings arise, gently allow them to be present and send them warmth and love also.

Now, imagine that the water line is now passing your eyebrows and then your cheeks, and send tenderness and loving-kindness to that area of your body. Now, allow your imagination to visualize the water level slowly passing down through the rest of your body. Try just to greet each body part, making time to pause and send loving-kindness to each area. If you notice any tension, try to meet these areas with tenderness.

Continue noticing the water level moving down through your body until there is no more water left. Take a moment to sit with whatever feelings or sensations are present. Nourish this moment for as long as you like.

Take a few deep breaths and open your eyes.

Giving and Receiving Compassion

There will always be times when you will find yourself hurting alongside other people who are hurting. All humans suffer. This is a part of life. The giving and receiving compassion meditation, developed by Neff and Germer (2018), allows you to practice sending compassion to yourself while also sending compassion to others. Unlike the loving-kindness meditation, the giving and receiving meditation practice will cultivate compassion through the breath instead of words and phrases. The following exercise comes from Neff and Germer's *Mindful Self-Compassion Workbook* (2018), and is used with permission.

Putting Your Skills into Practice

Sit comfortably, close your eyes, and if you like, put a hand over your heart or another soothing place as a reminder to bring not just awareness but loving awareness to your experience and to yourself.

Savoring the Breath

Take a few deep, relaxing breaths, noticing how your breath nourishes your body as you inhale and soothes your body as you exhale.

Now let your breath find its own natural rhythm. Continue feeling the sensation of breathing in and breathing out. If you like, allow yourself to be gently rocked and caressed by the rhythm of your breathing.

Warming Up Awareness

Now focus your attention on your inbreath, letting yourself savor the sensation of breathing in, noticing how your inbreath nourishes your body, breath after breath...and then release your breath.

As you breathe, begin to breathe in kindness and compassion for yourself. Just feel the quality of kindness and compassion as you breathe in, or if you prefer, letting a word or image ride on your inbreath.

Now shift your focus to your outbreath, feeling your body breathe out, feeling the ease of exhalation.

Please call to mind someone whom you love or someone who is struggling and needs compassion. Visualize that person clearly in your mind.

Begin directing your outbreath to this person, offering the ease of breathing out.

If you wish, send kindness and compassion to this person with each outbreath, one breath after another.

In for Me, Out for You

Now focus on the sensation of breathing both in and out, savoring the sensation of breathing in and out.

Begin breathing in for yourself and out for the other person. "In for me and out for you." "One for me and one for you." What do you need to feel safe and comfortable with others?

And as you breathe, draw kindness and compassion in for yourself and breathe kindness and compassion out for the other person.

If you wish, you can focus a little more on yourself ("Two for me and one for you") or the other person ("One for me and three for you"), or just let it be an equal flow—whatever feels right in the moment.

Let go of any unnecessary effort, allowing this meditation to be as easy as breathing.

Allow your breath to flow in and out, like the gentle movement of the ocean—a limitless, boundless flow—flowing in and flowing out. Let yourself be a part of this limitless, boundless flow. An ocean of compassion.

Gently open your eyes.

Reflection

In the space below, journal your response to the questions provided.

Were you able to receive the compassion you were offering to yourself?

_____

Who did you give compassion to in this meditation?

_____

Did you notice a difference between the giving and receiving of compassion? How did your body change when you shifted from giving to receiving?

_____

_____

Were you able to offer compassion to your obsessions? If not, what got in the way of you experimenting with offering compassion to your thoughts, images, sensations, feelings, and urges?

_____

_____

You Are More Than Your OCD: Valuing the Whole You

I believe that recognizing and valuing who you are outside your OCD is a crucial part of creating a solid self-compassion practice, as it helps you to acknowledge that you are more than the thoughts you have and more than your diagnosis. Oftentimes, OCD can become so loud and persuasive that it will make you believe that you are your OCD. Valuing the Whole You requires you to take stock of your goodness and your fine qualities that go unnoticed. Maybe they go unnoticed because you are so consumed with the content of your obsessions. Perhaps you avoid appreciating yourself in fear of being seen as "self-absorbed" or "bragging," or maybe you genuinely don't feel you have any qualities to celebrate. Hear me loud and clearly. You have *many* talents and gifts and unique characteristics. In the following pages, you will first identify your many qualities and values, and then you will be asked to practice a meditation in which you dive deeper into the practice of celebrating the goodness that is *you!*

Reflection

In the list below, circle as many qualities and traits about yourself as you can. Give yourself permission to circle qualities that you possess *sometimes*, but not all the time, as well as qualities you *used* to have. Try not to compare yourself to others; instead, simply take an inventory of abilities and talents you have or have had in the past.

Accepting	Hard-working	Persuasive	Sentimental
Adventurous	Honest	Playful	Sharing
Affectionate	Hopeful	Practical	Skillful
Ambitious	Humble	Protective	Sociable
Analytical	Humorous	Punctual	Spontaneous
Authentic	Imaginative	Rational	Sympathetic
Brave	Insightful	Realistic	Thorough
Caring	Intelligent	Reflective	Tidy
Cheerful	Kind	Relaxed	Tolerant
Comforting	Leader-like	Reliable	Trusting
Communicative	Loyal	Resilient	Understanding
Compassionate	Mature	Resourceful	Vivacious
Courageous	Modest	Respectful	Warm
Creative	Objective	Responsible	Well-rounded
Encouraging	Optimistic	Responsive	Wise
Enthusiastic	Organized	Romantic	Witty
Flexible	Passionate	Secure	Youthful
Forgiving	Patient	Self-reliant	_____
Friendly	Patriotic	Self-sufficient	_____
Genuine	Perceptive	Selfless	_____
Graceful	Personable	Sensitive	_____

Now, find a comfortable position, taking a few slow breaths in and out. Try to notice where you might be holding on to tension and slowly release any areas where you are clenching or tightening. Gently close your eyes and bring your awareness to your body.

Now, bring your attention to one of your qualities and take a moment to really savor that quality. If you can, really drop down into an experience of deep appreciation for having this quality. If you are struggling to identify any good qualities, maybe just appreciate your dedication to trying this meditation. With your breath still being soft and steady, if you can, try to really drop down into appreciating these qualities about yourself.

You may notice some discomfort and uneasiness with this meditation. This may be a practice that you have not done for some time, if ever. If you can, notice if self-judgment arises and try to stay with the experience of appreciation instead of moving back into self-judgment.

Now, try to bring to mind any specific people who took part in and helped you develop such qualities. Maybe it was a friend, a parent, or a teacher. Take some time and send that person appreciation also. Allow yourself just to enjoy and savor the experience of appreciating your good qualities.

Slowly, when you are ready, open your eyes.

Moving Forward: What Works for You?

Before you move into the rest of this workbook, I would first like you to reflect on your experience of practicing self-compassion—nonjudgmentally and compassionately, of course!

Self-Compassion Exercises Cheat Sheet

Like any new skill, you will need to remember to practice these self-compassion exercises throughout your OCD recovery. At the end of this chapter (after the Chapter Reflection below) is a cheat sheet of the different self-compassion practices you have learned in this chapter. You will find this cheat sheet helpful as you move throughout this workbook. I also strongly encourage you to go to this book's website (http://www.newharbinger.com/47766) to download a PDF copy of this cheat sheet for printing, to help you track over time which exercises are becoming more useful for you.

Chapter Reflection

What practices and meditations were my favorites?

_____

_____

Are there any practices I did not like? What modifications could I make?

_____

_____

Are there any practices that I feel I need to work on? What would help me?

_____

_____

What words or phrases resonated most with me?

_____

_____

How can I implement these practices into my daily life?

_____

_____

What will get in the way of my continued self-compassion practice?

_____

_____

Who can support me with my self-compassion practice?

_____

_____

My Self-Compassion Exercises

Self-Compassionate Practices	Reflection
Visualizing Your Compassionate Self	
The Language of Self-Compassion	
What Would My Compassionate Self Say?	
Taking a Self-Compassionate Break	
Nurturing Your Suffering with Physical Touch	
Compassionate Letter Writing	
RAIN	
Compassionate Friend Meditation	
Loving-Kindness Meditation	
Affectionate Breathing Meditation	
Compassionate Body Scan	
Giving and Receiving Meditation	
Appreciating My Good Qualities Meditation	

CHAPTER 4

Common Self-Compassion Roadblocks During Exposure and Response Prevention

All human beings struggle with self-compassion in some capacity. Many of us are brought up in cultures and family systems that promote self-deprecation as a form of motivation and self-restraint. Generally speaking, in the Western world, we highly value being humble and self-sufficient—pulling ourselves up by the bootstraps—and this impacts how we treat ourselves. When I was in my twenties, I worked for a company with a staff T-shirt that had "You can rest when you are dead" on the back in big, bold letters. I bet if you think back, you too can recollect the many faulty messages you received about how we deserve to be treated.

Individuals with OCD often have additional roadblocks practicing self-compassion in daily life and when practicing exposure and response prevention. In this chapter, you will identify your specific self-compassion roadblocks and reflect on ways to target these roadblocks using the concepts, practices, and tools learned in previous chapters.

Reflection

Using the checklist below, identify the common reasons you struggle with practicing self-compassion. Once you have filled out the checklist, the rest of this chapter will help you create new beliefs and practices around these roadblocks so that you can get the most out of the ERP exercises in this workbook. Examples of how Simone, Tanya, Todd, and Alex worked through their roadblocks are also provided throughout this chapter. If your specific roadblock to self-compassion is not included, please enter it in the space provided.

Common OCD-Related Roadblocks to Practicing Mindful Self-Compassion

☐ I do not deserve self-compassion because of the content of my obsessions.

☐ I am not worthy of self-compassion because I have a mental illness.

☐ I am too preoccupied with anxiety, panic, and uncertainty to practice self-compassion.

☐ It feels wrong to practice self-compassion.

☐ Self-criticism and self-punishment are how I motivate myself.

☐ What if self-compassion makes me weak or lazy?

☐ What if practicing self-compassion makes me snap or lose control?

☐ Practicing self-compassion could make me self-centered.

☐ Other: _____

☐ Other: _____

Roadblock 1   *I do not deserve self-compassion because of the content of my thoughts.*

Simone   Simone was quick to reject the idea of practicing self-compassion: "I am an awful human being. There is no way I can practice self-compassion. I don't deserve nice things. I don't deserve to be treated well. My thoughts are too horrendous!" Simone felt that she must be punished for her thoughts and urges and attributed her worth to these thoughts.

Believing that the content of your obsessions disqualifies you from deserving self-compassion is one of the most common self-compassion roadblocks. People with OCD tend to label themselves as "bad," "wrong," or with other shame-filled words because they believe that their thoughts directly reflect their values and morals. This expectation is where things go terribly wrong. All humans have strange, dark, intrusive thoughts. Just because you have strange thoughts does not mean you get demoted to "bad human." Just because you feel a sensation or urge that confuses or repels you does not mean you no longer deserve respect and compassion.

When you label yourself as "bad" or "wrong" because of your thoughts, feelings, images, sensations, and urges, not only will you be more likely to treat yourself poorly, you also are more likely to accept being treated poorly by others. The core thing to remember here is that your worth as a human being has *nothing* (and I repeat, nothing) to do with the thoughts or images you experience or the feelings, sensations, or urges you feel. *All* humans deserve respect and compassion, and you are not exempt from this because of the obsessions you experience.

Putting Your Skills into Practice: Correcting Faulty Thoughts

Faulty belief: "I do not deserve self-compassion because of the content of my obsessions."

Using the section below, write a strong alternative thought that you find helpful when managing this faulty thought.

Simone's Alternative Thought: "There is no thought or feeling that disqualifies me from being worthy of self-compassion. My obsessions do not define me. I am a human being, and every human deserves kindness, care, and respect."

_____

_____

_____

What core self-compassion concepts (from chapter 2) or self-compassion practices (from chapter 3) might help you manage this particular roadblock?

_____

_____

_____

Roadblock 2   *I am not worthy of self-compassion because I have a mental illness.*

Tanya   When Tanya came to see me, she had no idea what was happening to her. No one in her family had a mental illness that she knew of, and she grew up with a strong family assumption that people with mental illnesses are weak. At first, Tanya was relieved to be diagnosed with OCD, because it helped her understand what was happening to her. However, very quickly, Tanya went back to beating herself up for having a mental illness:

"I am a broken human being." "There is something wrong with me." "I am unlovable because of my OCD."

As Tanya and I discussed mental health stigma, I asked, "I wonder what you would say if one of your kids came to you and said they had OCD? How might you act toward them?"

Tanya took some time to think about this and replied, "I would hug them and tell them I will help them."

"I can see what a compassionate mother you are!" I said. "You didn't judge or condemn them. I wonder if you could offer that same kindness and tenderness to yourself? I wonder if you could lead by example and teach our next generation that people who have mental illnesses have nothing to be ashamed of and that people with mental illnesses deserve to be treated equally, with respect? Would you be interested in possibly taking on that role in your family?"

Tanya nodded. After some thought, she sat up on the couch and said, "I never want my children to have to hide their struggles from me. I want them to know that it's okay to have mental health problems. I was never given that opportunity, and it has made this so much harder to bear."

One of the biggest reasons we struggle with self-compassion is the stigma of having a mental illness. Still, to this day, despite some improvements, society still grossly misunderstands what it means to have a mental illness, especially OCD. If we look back at history, we can track the stigma of mental illness being the result of lack of education about mental illnesses, the unwillingness to be correctly informed about mental illnesses, and the absence of open-mindedness. The stigma of mental illness is unwillingly taught to us from an early age, but this false narrative can be untaught.

Forgive me while I speak frankly, but whether you buy into this nonsense about people with mental illness being "less than" is entirely up to you. As you have learned already in this workbook, your worth has *nothing* to do with the thoughts you have, the feelings you experience, the behaviors you engage in, or the diagnosis you were given. Having a mental illness is not a choice and it is *not* your fault that you have OCD. You are worthy of self-compassion, no matter what mental health struggles you have.

In fact, self-compassion is the act of treating yourself kindly when enduring a difficult moment or situation. You know more than anyone that those with mental illnesses come with countless difficult situations and painful moments. If you are in pain—whether the source is medical, physical, spiritual, or mental—your pain is worthy of self-compassion.

Putting Your Skills into Practice: Correcting Faulty Thoughts

Faulty thought or belief: "I do not deserve self-compassion because I have a mental illness/es."

Using the section below, write an alternative thought that you find helpful when managing this faulty thought.

Tanya's Alternate Thought: "Having a mental illness does not disqualify me from being treated with respect and compassion. We can't just give ourselves self-compassion when things are going well. We must also practice self-compassion when things are tough, and when we are struggling."

_____

_____

_____

Is there a core self-compassion concept or self-compassion practice that might help you manage this particular roadblock?

_____

_____

_____

Roadblock 3   *I am too preoccupied with anxiety, panic, and uncertainty even to consider self-compassion.*

Todd   Todd reported that one of the biggest reasons he struggled to use his self-compassion skills was his preoccupation with uncertainty, anxiety, and panic symptoms: "I just get so lost in my thoughts that I completely forget that self-compassion is even an option. To be honest, I sometimes lose complete sense of time and space, and I don't even notice it until hours later."

Becoming *mindful* of your experience of anxiety, uncertainty, and doubt will be important as you move throughout this workbook and throughout your recovery. Your ability to be aware of your anxiety in your body will allow you to choose to move toward self-compassion instead of toward compulsive safety-seeking behaviors. If you find that you are on autopilot, responding to fear with resistance all day, try to bring your attention to what *is* happening in this moment. Slow down and make an intentional effort to lean into your discomfort. This will involve your becoming an observer to your experience of anxiety. Instead of saying, "I am anxious," say, "I am noticing anxiety in my body." If you notice an intrusive feeling, sensation, or urge appear in your body, slow down and make space for this discomfort to rise and fall on its own, nonjudgmentally. If you are being barraged with an onslaught of intrusive thoughts and images, practice observing them like clouds in the sky. Watch them without engaging in their content. Once you have become aware of your preoccupation with anxiety, you can then choose to direct your attention toward kindness and warmth for yourself.

Putting Your Skills into Practice: Correcting Faulty Thoughts

Faulty thought or belief: "I am too preoccupied with anxiety, panic, and uncertainty even to consider self-compassion."

Using the section below, write an alternative thought that you find helpful when managing this faulty thought.

Todd's Alternative Thought: "With practice, I can learn to slow down and become more aware of the present moment. I can work toward being aware of the anxiety in my body and lean into those sensations with self-compassion instead of being preoccupied with my obsessions."

_____

_____

_____

What core self-compassion concepts or self-compassion practices might help you manage this particular roadblock?

_____

_____

_____

Roadblock 4   _It feels wrong to practice self-compassion._

Alex   Alex mentioned multiple times that it felt wrong to practice self-compassion: "I feel like I am irresponsible and a bad person unless I am giving fear my attention."

There is a common cognitive distortion called "emotional reasoning." Emotional reasoning is an error in our thinking that involves us believing that if we feel something, that feeling must be true or a fact. I brought to Alex's attention that he was avoiding self-compassion, along with many of his emotions, simply because of a feeling he had. Just because he felt "wrong" or "irresponsible" does not mean he *is* wrong or irresponsible.

The work of managing OCD involves being uncertain. Uncertainty and willingness to be uncomfortable is the cornerstone of your ERP practices. Alex had to accept being uncertain instead of assuming that the feelings were the facts. With practice, Alex learned how to observe this feeling of "wrongness" and allow it to be present and meet whatever discomfort he felt with kindness and tenderness. It can "feel real," but that does not mean it is true. Remember, we don't want to invalidate your experience. But we do want to be sure we are responding to thoughts and feelings with wisdom and in ways that bring us to long-term recovery.

Putting Your Skills into Practice: Correcting Faulty Thoughts

Faulty Thought: "It feels wrong to practice self-compassion."

Using the section below, write an alternative thought that you find helpful when managing this faulty thought.

Alex's Alternate Thought: "Just because something feels wrong does not mean it is wrong. I am allowed to be kind to myself, even when things feel wrong. I will not allow the presence of a feeling, even if it is painfully uncomfortable, to determine how I respond or how I treat myself."

_____

_____

_____

What core self-compassion concepts or self-compassion practices might help you manage this particular roadblock?

_____

_____

_____

Roadblock 5   *Self-criticism and self-punishment are how I motivate myself.*

Simone   Simone had strong beliefs around the role self-criticism played in her life: "Being hard on myself keeps me in check. It's how I keep myself motivated. The harder on myself I am, the more successful I become."

Our society has extreme views on motivation. Many people, but especially those with OCD, believe that self-criticism and self-punishment are their best ways of holding themselves accountable and staying motivated. Maybe you, too, believe that to accomplish anything, you must somehow threaten yourself with all the serious consequences that might occur if you don't perform well. Thankfully, however, we have the science to prove that this is not true at all. A study by Williams, Stark, and Foster (2008) found that people who practice self-compassion end up procrastinating less and have lower anticipatory anxiety levels. Research has also shown that students who practice self-compassion are more likely to try again after not performing well or even failing at a task (Neely et al. 2009). Lastly, research has shown that people who show high levels of self-criticism and self-punishment are much more susceptible to developing obsessive-compulsive disorder or generalized anxiety disorder (Sugiura and Fisak 2019).

Putting Your Skills into Practice: Correcting Faulty Thoughts

Faulty Thought: *"Self-criticism and self-punishment are how I motivate myself."*

Using the section below, write an alternative thought that you find helpful when managing this faulty thought.

Simone's Alternative Thought: "Scientific evidence shows that self-criticism is not an effective motivator. Even if it gets me to do a task, I end up feeling terrible afterward. There is more evidence proving that long-term motivation increases with the practice of self-compassion."

_____

_____

_____

What core self-compassion concepts or self-compassion practices might help you manage this particular roadblock?

_____

_____

_____

Roadblock 6   *What if self-compassion makes me weak or lazy?*

Todd   When I suggested to Todd that he practice self-compassion alongside his ERP, Todd listened but quickly shook his head. He replied, "Let's be real! Self-compassion makes people weak and lazy, and I refuse to lose everything I have worked for just so that I can be kind to myself."

My eyebrows raised as I heard this. "Todd, is this how you talk to yourself every day?"

Todd chuckled. "I am dead serious. Being self-compassionate is like admitting to weakness, and I cannot afford to be weak. I have worked too hard to get to where I am!"

There is a big misconception that self-compassion is merely lying on the couch, licking your wounds, and dwelling on how hard life is. This could not be further from the truth. In my humble opinion, practicing self-compassion is one of the most courageous, badass actions you can take when you are suffering. Also, practicing self-compassion is significantly more effective than the safety behaviors you might engage in, such as avoidance, thought suppression, self-criticism, and self-punishment. Instead, choose to stand up to fear with dignity, respect, and self-worth. Instead of engaging in self-criticism and self-punishment simply because you fear becoming weak or lazy, stare the fear of becoming weak and lazy right in the face and choose kindness and tenderness. There is nothing "weak" about that.

It is also essential that you examine your beliefs about productivity, as they can keep you in a cycle of "busy-ness." You might find that you engage in compulsive productivity. This is not only exhausting and ineffective; it also feeds the faulty belief that you are worthy only when you are running yourself ragged. You may also find that your compulsive drive for productivity is so exhausting and anxiety provoking that you are then unable to complete what you originally set out to achieve. The result: you beat yourself up even more. It is a vicious cycle. Hear me loud and clear here: there is nothing impressive about being busy all the time. Please stop trying to convince yourself that you are more worthy just because you are productive. While it is true that productivity is essential to our daily functioning, these fears and faulty beliefs become incredibly problematic when they prevent you from meeting your emotional and physical needs. Learn to listen to your body and respect it when it tells you to rest.

Putting Your Skills into Practice: Correcting Faulty Thoughts

Faulty Thought: "Being self-compassionate might make me weak or lazy."

Using the section below, write an alternative thought that you find helpful when managing this faulty thought.

Todd's Alternative Thought: "Practicing self-compassion has nothing to do with being weak or lazy. Self-compassion is a practice of meeting our pain with tenderness while engaging in life and taking care of our well-being. Both can be done at the same time."

_____

_____

_____

What core self-compassion concepts or self-compassion practices might help you manage this particular roadblock?

_____

_____

_____

Roadblock 7   *What if practicing self-compassion makes me snap or lose control?*

Alex   During one of our sessions together, I asked Alex if he would be willing to practice a self-compassion exercise to help him hold space for the discomfort that arises while working on his self-compassionate ERP exercises. Alex was hesitant and explained that he was afraid that practicing self-kindness might cause him to "snap" and "lose control" of his mind and actions. Alex felt it was necessary to stay hyper-focused on his thoughts and behaviors all day, in case he lost control of himself and harmed someone.

This fear is pervasive for those who experience OCD, especially for (but not limited to) those who struggle with harm obsessions, sexual orientation obsessions, relationship obsessions, pedophilia and sexual obsessions, moral obsessions, and emotional contamination obsessions. In this case, the person is compulsively avoiding self-compassion in fear that these practices might cause them to let down their guard and do something "unforgivable" or "unrepairable."

If you, too, find that you need to hyper-control your behavior, please remember that this only reinforces your fears and makes it harder to break the cycle of obsessions and compulsions. You must use your self-compassion practices as an opportunity to meet your fear and uncertainty willingly and nonjudgmentally. This practice helped Alex understand the extent to which he tried to control his mind and behavior and how problematic and time-consuming it was for him.

Your recovery depends on your willingness to practice letting go of control. Taking this plunge into the practices of courage and compassion is a wonderful opportunity to do just that. You might benefit by employing the phrase, "Maybe I will, maybe I won't! Either way, I am going to practice being uncertain and compassionate, no matter what."

Putting Your Skills into Practice: Correcting Faulty Thoughts

Faulty Thought: "What if practicing self-compassion makes me snap or lose control?"

Using the section below, write a strong alternative thought that you find helpful when managing this faulty thought.

Alex's Alternative Thought: "The most crucial component of exposure and response prevention is tolerating uncertainty and leaning into things that trigger these fears. Practicing self-compassion is a great way to experience being uncertain and to improve my relationship with myself and my fears. I am going to face this fear and be kind to myself as I go."

_____

_____

_____

What core self-compassion concepts or self-compassion practices might help you manage this particular roadblock?

_____

_____

_____

Roadblock 8 *Practicing self-compassion might make me self-centered.*

Tanya   After learning about self-compassion, Tanya raised the concern that the practice of self-compassion would cause her to "swing too far" and become grandiose and egotistical. Tanya said she has a friend at work who was always bragging about herself, and she said she would never allow herself to become like that. Tanya asked, "Will treating myself with compassion cause me to become self-centered or narcissistic?"

Tanya's question is an excellent example of a common cognitive distortion called black-and-white thinking. Black-and-white thinking, also known as all-or-nothing thinking, involves thinking only in extremes. People who struggle with black-and-white thinking often see things as only one way or another, and they cannot imagine or tolerate a gray area in between. In this case, Tanya avoided the practice of self-compassion in fear that if she let go of self-criticism and treated herself with self-compassion, she would swing to the other end of the spectrum and become self-centered. The point to remember here is that things rarely exist at either end of a spectrum. There is often fluidity, and your work is to accept and make room for that fluidity. Once again, practice being uncertain and being present. Let's agree to worry about being self-centered only *if* that happens—and not a moment before. Until then, spread radical self-compassion into your world. Compassion is *not* egotistical or selfish, and *if* it becomes that, it is likely you were not practicing self-compassion at all.

As you move throughout this workbook, please become aware of your black-and-white thinking. Engaging in these cognitive distortions can often increase the chances of reacting to an obsession compulsively. Throughout your OCD recovery, you might find it helpful to note down when you became aware of black-and-white thinking and then, once again, tolerate the uncertainty and lean into that experience with self-compassion. This perfectly complements the work you will be doing with exposure and response prevention and will help you become aware of how black-and-white thinking interferes with your self-compassion practices.

Putting Your Skills into Practice: Correcting Faulty Thoughts

Faulty Thought: "Practicing self-compassion might make me self-centered."

Using the section on the following page, write a powerful alternative thought that you find helpful when managing this faulty thought.

Tanya's Alternative Thought: "I can practice self-compassion and learn that there are many ways to incorporate self-compassion without making the focus be on my own sense of importance. I am choosing to live in the gray area instead of black-and-white thinking."

_____

_____

_____

What core self-compassion concepts or self-compassion practices might help you manage this particular roadblock?

_____

_____

_____

Other Roadblocks

Please address any other roadblocks that you experience that were not discussed explicitly in this chapter in the journal section below.

Putting Your Skills into Practice: Correcting Faulty Thoughts

Faulty Thought: _____

Using the section below, come up with a strong, supportive alternative thought that may help you manage this roadblock (see other roadblocks for inspiration).

_____

_____

_____

What core self-compassion concepts or self-compassion practices might help you manage this particular roadblock?

_____

_____

_____

Putting Your Skills into Practice: Correcting Faulty Thoughts/Beliefs

Faulty Thought: _____

Using the section below, come up with a strong, supportive alternative thought that may help you manage this roadblock (see other roadblocks for inspiration).

_____

_____

_____

What core self-compassion concepts (from chapter two) or self-compassion practices (from chapter three) might help you manage this particular roadblock?

_____

_____

_____

PART TWO

Leaning into Fear and Uncertainty with Self-Compassion

Dear courageous one,

Congratulations on getting this far! You obviously value your wellness very much.

In part 2, you will learn how to lean into fear and uncertainty using self-compassion and exposure and response prevention. As you practice staring your fear right in the face, be prepared for your mind to shout, "Be careful!" or "You won't be able to handle this!" These thoughts will tempt you to return to engaging in compulsions to remove your discomfort. In response, there is one simple yet powerful sentence that I would like you to use each and every day. This sentence is...

It is a beautiful day to do hard things!

I say this to my patients every day and, I am now saying it directly to you, because it is true. You can do hard things! I know this because you have already done many, many hard things. And human beings are incredibly resilient. Now, it is essential to understand that your recovery is not going to be a linear process. You will have ups, and you will have downs. However, by doing one hard thing and then another, you will start to believe in yourself again. You will learn that you can tolerate high levels of uncertainty, fear, and discomfort without saying unkind words to yourself or treating yourself unkindly.

So, dear friend, pull your shoulders back, and put your hand on your heart, and do not give up. It's a beautiful day to do hard things!

Kimberley

CHAPTER 5

Identifying Your Obsessions and Compulsions

Before we begin practicing ERP, we need to do a thorough inventory of your obsessions and compulsions and prepare your ERP Challenge List—a list of all of the exposures you plan to engage in throughout this workbook. I like to call it an ERP Challenge List because I want you to think of it as just that: a list of challenges! Your ERP Challenge List is not a boring list of things you have to do, like a to-do list of your daily errands. Instead, the ERP Challenge List is a list of challenges that will help you stare your obsessions right in the eyes and take your life back from OCD. In this chapter, Alex will walk alongside you and give examples of his obsessions and compulsions. At the end of the chapter, Alex, Tanya, Todd, and Simone will provide examples of their ERP Challenge Lists.

Something to Consider

Some people with OCD find it triggering to document their obsessions and compulsions, as it triggers their perfectionism obsessions or other obsessions. In fact, these exercises may be considered an exposure in and of itself. As you follow the prompts provided in this chapter, do your best to allow for imperfection and uncertainty. Use these exercises as an opportunity to practice willingly and warmly nurturing whatever discomfort it induces. If you are really struggling, possibly ask a friend, family member, or trained mental health professional to sit with you as you fill out the provided prompts.

Identifying Your Obsessions

In this workbook, I have organized your obsessions into five main categories: intrusive thoughts, intrusive images, intrusive feelings, intrusive sensations, and intrusive urges. You may experience one, some, or all of these types of obsessions to varying degrees. Try to practice not comparing yourself to others or judging yourself negatively for the obsessions that you experience. If you do notice that you are responding critically, immediately employ the self-compassion practices and mindfulness skills you have learned in previous chapters. Remember, *it is a beautiful day to do hard things!* As you identify your specific intrusive thoughts, try not to get caught up in the content of these thoughts and what these thoughts mean about you. As you identify the obsessions you experience, practice being an observer of how these thoughts pull you into the O-C cycle.

Intrusive Thoughts

All humans experience intrusive thoughts. An intrusive thought is a thought that is unwanted and repetitive and that causes a significant degree of anxiety, uncertainty, and doubt. Intrusive thoughts can arise when exposed to a feared object, place, or internal trigger, or they may simply appear in your mind for no reason at all. Intrusive thoughts often present themselves as single words, single phrases, or sentences that commonly start with "What if." An intrusive thought can also be experienced in the form of a memory. Intrusive memories are thoughts focused on events that may or may not have occurred in the past, resulting in overwhelming uncertainty about what is real and what is not.

Reflection

In the space below, write down the intrusive thoughts you have experienced in the last two weeks. Try not to overwhelm yourself with too many details about your intrusive thoughts. We will have lots of opportunities during the exposure portion of this workbook to flesh out the specifics of your intrusive thoughts. For now, just write the most common intrusive thoughts. If you need more space, feel free to use a notepad, a journal, or a computer program to document your intrusive thoughts.

Alex's Intrusive Thought List

- "Kill."

- "Stab."

- "Murderer."

- "What if I want to hurt my students?"

- "What if snap in the middle of a lesson and go crazy?"

- "What if I am a pedophile?"

_____

_____

_____

_____

_____

_____

_____

_____

Intrusive Images

An intrusive image is a type of intrusive thought. Consider an intrusive image like a polaroid snapshot of a future or past event that you see in your mind. These intrusive images are unwanted and often explicit and distressing. They may appear randomly; when you come into contact with a feared object, place, or person; or when you experience internal triggers, such as sensations, thoughts, or other obsessions.

Reflection

Using the space below, list the intrusive images you experience. Again, do not feel you have to go into great detail, as you will have many opportunities to go into much greater detail later in this workbook.

Alex's Intrusive Image List

- Students on their knees, screaming.

- Students running from me in the school parking lot as I ruthlessly try to grab them.

- Sexually assaulting a student.

- Blood splashing across the floor.

- Carefully putting a gun and a knife into my school briefcase.

_____

_____

_____

_____

_____

_____

_____

_____

_____

Intrusive Feelings

A feeling is an emotional state, a consciousness of sensations, or a general bodily awareness. An intrusive feeling is a emotion or experience that is repetitive, unwanted, and causes significant distress, anxiety, and panic. Common examples of intrusive feelings include guilt, "not right" feelings, the feeling of impending doom, derealization, depersonalization, and disgust.

Derealization is an experience in which a person feels detached from their surroundings and feels as if their experiences are not real. Depersonalization is an experience in which a person feels like they are detached from their own body, as if they are looking down on themselves from above, or as an outside observer of one's actions. Derealization and depersonalization cause significant distress and can impair functioning.

Another common intrusive feeling is the feeling of disgust—the feeling of revulsion and disapproval related to an object, person, or action that is perceived as offensive or unpleasant. An individual with contamination obsessions may have predominantly disgust obsessions. In this case, their obsession does not involve the fear of being contaminated by dirt or germs, but instead, the fear and aversion to the feeling of disgust. We will discuss how to manage disgust in much greater detail in chapter 11.

Guilt is a common intrusive feeling, especially for those whose obsessions are related to behavior that does not align with their values, morals, or beliefs. Guilt is a normal emotional response when you have behaved in a way you hadn't planned or don't approve of. However, people with OCD often feel guilt at levels that are grossly disproportionate to their actions. For this reason, guilt can be conceptualized as an obsession, as it triggers repetitive cycles of anxiety, uncertainty, and doubt, causing the person with OCD to engage in safety-seeking compulsions to remove the experience of guilt. The management of guilt is also addressed in much greater detail in chapter 11.

Reflection

Using the space below, list the intrusive feelings you have experienced in the past two weeks.

Alex's List of Intrusive Feelings

- intrusive feelings of guilt
- derealization

_____

_____

_____

_____

_____

_____

_____

_____

_____

Intrusive Sensations

An intrusive sensation is a sensation, physical perception, or experience that is repetitive and disturbing and causes significant distress to one's daily life. While intrusive sensations may include any physical sensation, some common intrusive sensations related to OCD and anxiety include dizziness, shortness of breath, nausea, shaking, blinking, the urge to urinate or defecate, light-headedness, an irregular heartbeat, a lump in the throat, and numbness.

All humans with anxiety experience some degree of intrusive sensations. However, intrusive sensations are particularly difficult for those with obsessions such as sensorimotor obsessions or health anxiety obsessions and for those who experience panic attacks. People with sensorimotor OCD tend to be hyperaware of their intrusive sensations and spend a great deal of time checking to see if their intrusive sensations are present or not. For those who experience health anxiety, intrusive sensations can be very triggering. In these cases, anxiety symptoms can be misinterpreted as severe, imminent health conditions, causing the person to then have a heightened anxiety response. This corresponding anxiety then causes them to have even more intrusive sensations, and they can get stuck in a vicious cycle of anxiety.

A common intrusive sensation for individuals with sexual obsessions is sexual arousal. You may notice sexual arousal at times that greatly confuse and alarm you. In this case, you may question the meaning and intention behind the arousing sensations, causing you to engage in compulsive checking, reassurance seeking, or mental rumination. These compulsions often cause hyperawareness of arousal, increasing the intensity and frequency of the sensation of arousal.

Reflection

Using the space below, list any intrusive sensations you try to avoid. Also, include the specific sensations of anxiety that you feel when you are triggered.

Alex's Intrusive Sensation List

- shortness of breath

- dizziness

- chest tightness

- sexual arousal

_____

_____

_____

_____

_____

_____

_____

_____

_____

_____

Intrusive Urges

An intrusive urge is an experience where one feels an intense impulse to engage in an action or behave in a particular way. These intrusive urges are incredibly disturbing because they do not line up with the person's beliefs and morals. These intrusive urges, similar to intrusive feelings, can be very hard to describe and can make people with OCD question their own intentions, morals, and capabilities.

Reflection

Using the space below, list the intrusive urges you experience.

Alex's Intrusive Urge List

- The urge to stab a student.

- The urge to hold a student down.

- The urge to act aggressively toward a student.

_____

_____

_____

_____

_____

_____

_____

_____

Identifying Your Compulsions

You will now identify the specific compulsive safety behaviors you use to decrease or eliminate the anxiety, uncertainty, and doubt related to your obsessions. There are hundreds of different compulsive behaviors. However, for simplicity, I have organized the most common into ten main categories. You may find that your compulsions fall into some or all of these categories. Once again, there is no right or wrong presentation of OCD.

As you continue with this inventory, give yourself as much respect and compassion as you can while honestly reflecting on your safety-seeking compulsions. If your specific compulsion is not listed, please don't be alarmed. The below categories and their examples are simply a guide to help you gather the information you need to create your own personalized ERP Challenge List.

Avoidant Compulsions

Avoidant compulsions are safety behaviors that involve the act of removing yourself from people, places, or objects that trigger your obsession. There is no limit to what you can avoid. I encourage you to document the activities, people, physical items, and places you avoid throughout your day to avoid being triggered.

Reflection

Using the space below, list all of the avoidant compulsions you have engaged in over the last two weeks.

_____

_____

_____

_____

_____

_____

_____

_____

Checking Compulsions

Checking compulsions are safety behaviors done to ensure that you are not responsible for a catastrophe and that danger or consequences will not occur to yourself and others. Some common examples of physical checking compulsions include checking stoves and other appliances, locks, electrical outlets, hair straighteners, windows, and pillboxes. Checking compulsions can also be done only in your head—mentally examining and inspecting particular objects, people, personal sensations, and emotions to remove your uncertainty and distress.

Reflection

Using the space below, list all of the checking compulsions you have engaged in over the last two weeks.

_____

_____

_____

_____

_____

_____

_____

_____

Cleansing Compulsions

Cleansing compulsions are behaviors done to remove anxiety, uncertainty, and disgust related to fears of contamination, illness, or death. Cleansing compulsions are common for those with contamination obsessions but can also be related to other subtypes of OCD, such as emotional contamination, health anxiety, "just right," and moral obsessions. Cleansing compulsions can be done to remove actual contaminants or to remove the feeling of being contaminated. Common cleansing compulsions include hand washing, showering, tidying, changing clothing, or compulsive grooming.

Reflection

Using the space below, list all of the cleansing compulsions you have engaged in over the last two weeks.

_____

_____

_____

_____

_____

_____

_____

_____

Compulsive Counting

Counting compulsions involve mentally or verbally repeating numbers or performing actions in multiples. Counting compulsions are often done to neutralize a behavior done a "bad" number of times or neutralize or avoid another obsession. A person who engages in counting compulsions might count their actions (such as how many times they turn on the lights) or count during a behavior (such as counting to four repetitively while brushing their teeth). Compulsive counting can often involve counting to "good" or "safe" numbers or avoiding specific "taboo" or "bad" numbers such as 13, 666, or others, depending on the person's beliefs or superstitions. Compulsive counting may also be at random, particularly for those who have "not just right" obsessions.

Reflection

Using the space below, list all of the counting compulsions you have engaged in over the last two weeks.

_____

_____

_____

_____

_____

_____

_____

_____

_____

Compulsive Prayer

Compulsive prayer is a repetitive or ritualized form of prayer performed to ensure that the prayer was done correctly, purely, and with good intent. Compulsive prayer is also commonly done to undo perceived "bad" behaviors or thoughts that go against one's religion or spiritual beliefs. Compulsive prayer also involves repetitive reciting of religious texts and devotions.

Reflection

Using the space below, list all of the prayer-related compulsions you have engaged in over the last two weeks.

_____

_____

_____

_____

_____

_____

_____

_____

_____

Hoarding

Hoarding is now considered its own disorder, with its own diagnosis, and is no longer classified as a form of obsessive-compulsive disorder. However, people with obsessive-compulsive disorder commonly engage in compulsive hoarding. Compulsive hoarding involves keeping and storing objects in fear that they may be needed. Hoarded items may be sentimental in nature or could be miscellaneous and meaningless objects, such as receipts, plastic bags, or lists. Hoarding compulsions also involve mental hoarding, which includes mentally preserving or neutralizing an emotion, feeling, or experience. Mental hoarding also involves hoarding memories in the hope of keeping them safe or in case they will be needed at a later time for reassurance.

Reflection

Using the space below, list all of the hoarding compulsions you have engaged in over the last two weeks.

_____

_____

_____

_____

_____

_____

_____

_____

_____

Mental Compulsions

Mental compulsions involve rumination and intellectual reflection on past and possible future experiences. These compulsions take many forms, but they are often explained as "mental gymnastics" or "solving," done to forecast, correct, or find meaning in any specific uncertainties one may have. Mental compulsions often involve scrutinizing one's past or future intentions, previously made decisions, and alternative outcomes to events that have already taken place. Mental compulsions often sound like, "Could X happen? Would I want X to happen? What would be the consequence if X does happen? What would I do if X happened? How can I prevent X from happening?" For example, Alex listed, "(1) try to mentally solve if I want to hurt or sexually assault my students, (2) try to figure out if I enjoyed hearing about the teacher who harmed his students, (3) reviewing past interactions with students to see if I was attracted to them, (4) mentally rehearsing what I will say and how I will act so I don't snap and hurt them."

Reflection

Using the space below, list all of the mental compulsions you have engaged in over the last two weeks.

_____

_____

_____

_____

_____

_____

_____

_____

Movement and Touching Compulsions

Movement and touching compulsions involve moving or touching any object or body part to reduce the experience of anxiety, uncertainty, or another form of discomfort. Movement and touching compulsions may also be done to achieve a sense of symmetry or attain the "right" feeling. Some examples of movement or touching compulsions include repetitively touching personal or household items, moving books or pencils or other objects on your desk, or shifting one's own posture until the experience of uncertainty or discomfort decreases or ceases. Please note that it is not uncommon for movement or touching compulsions to include counting or other neutralizing compulsions. Feel free to list these compulsions in whatever section feels most appropriate.

Reflection

Using the space below, list all of the movement or touching compulsions you have engaged in over the last two weeks.

_____

_____

_____

_____

_____

_____

_____

_____

Neutralizing Compulsions

Neutralizing compulsions are safety-seeking behaviors that "undo" or reverse negative thoughts, feelings, sensations, images, and urges. These compulsions can be done physically or mentally. Physical neutralizing compulsions involve performing any action or having any thought that is perceived as positive to neutralize or remove one's discomfort, uncertainty, or the possibility of one's perceived negative outcomes. Examples of neutralizing compulsions include restarting or reopening computer applications or programs, moving an item left if it was first moved right (or vice versa), reversing one's actions back to the original position, walking back through hallways or doorways, and replacing obsessions with "positive" or "good" thoughts.

Reflection

Using the space below, list all of the neutralizing compulsions you have engaged in over the last two weeks.

_____

_____

_____

_____

_____

_____

_____

_____

Reassurance Seeking

Reassurance-seeking compulsions involve pursuing certainty through others to reduce one's own discomfort, uncertainty, or doubt. Reassurance seeking can be done in multiple ways. A person with OCD might seek reassurance by asking another person an obsession-related question to remove uncertainty or state an obsession-related fact to see if others disagree or agree with one's stance or concern on the topic. Reassurance seeking can also be performed by explaining their obsession to a family member or loved one and then watching their loved one's reaction to see if they are concerned or not. Reassurance-seeking compulsions also involve using internet search engines, books, podcasts, and online articles to remove or reduce one's experiences of uncertainty and doubt about the obsession.

Reflection

Using the space below, list all of the reassurance-seeking compulsions you have engaged in over the last two weeks.

_____

_____

_____

_____

_____

_____

_____

_____

Self-Punishment

Self-punishment is done not to reduce uncertainty but to discipline yourself for your thoughts, feelings, sensations, urges, and compulsive behaviors. In most cases, people with OCD perform self-punishment compulsions hoping that punishing themselves will decrease the occurrence of obsessions or decrease or prevent compulsions in the future. Self-punishment includes acts of self-criticism, self-blame, self-harm, avoidance of self-care, and withholding pleasure.

Reflection

Using the space below, list all of the self-punishment compulsions you have engaged in over the last two weeks.

_____

_____

_____

_____

_____

_____

_____

_____

_____

Treatment-Related Compulsions

Compulsions can find their way into any part of your life, and treatment and recovery are no exception. As you move through the following chapters, you might observe the inclination to return to some mindfulness, self-compassion, or ERP exercises *with repetition and urgency,* as they provide some degree of relief from fear, uncertainty, and doubt. Examples of this include:

- Engaging in an exposure to prove that you do not enjoy or approve of your obsession.

- Engaging in an exposure, such as flooding and scriptwriting, to disprove your obsession will happen.

- For people with the OCD subtype of obsessing about obsessing, engaging in exposures to prove they are getting better or performing treatment properly to remove the uncertainty that they might be getting worse.

- Using self-compassion to justify avoidance. In this case, self-compassion is unintentionally used to justify *not* facing one's fear. (Example: "It's okay. You don't have to do that exposure. Not doing this exposure is the kind thing to do.")

- Correcting faulty thoughts to reduce the uncertainty that feared events will occur.

- Compulsively over-reading OCD literature to reassure yourself that your obsessions are common and not a reflection on you as a person.

Reflection

Using the space below, list all of the treatment-related compulsions you have engaged in over the last two weeks.

_____

_____

_____

_____

_____

_____

_____

Reflection

Well, that was a big task! Let's first take a moment to congratulate yourself on a job well done! Before we move on, let's do a quick check-in. In the space below, reflect on the questions provided.

As you wrote down your lists of obsessions and compulsions, how did you treat yourself? Did you criticize yourself in any way? Did you encourage or discourage yourself during this process?

_____

_____

_____

Many with OCD are hard on themselves as they do an inventory on their obsessions and compulsions. What self-compassion tools and practices might be helpful for you at this time?

_____

_____

_____

Creating Your ERP Challenge List

Now, using the list of obsessions and compulsions you identified earlier in this chapter, you will create your ERP Challenge List—the blueprint you will use every day to help you plan and implement your exposures with effective response prevention.

Reflection

Now it is time for you to document all of the ways you can expose yourself to your obsessions. Go back and reflect on your lists of obsessions and compulsions earlier in this chapter and use the prompts provided below to help you identify as many opportunities for future exposures as you can.

- What events or activities trigger your obsessions?

- What events or activities do you avoid in fear of being triggered?

- Are there any people who trigger your intrusive thoughts, images, sensations, feelings, or urges? If so, what specifically do they do that triggers you?

- Are there any people you avoid in fear of being triggered?

- Are there any places that trigger your obsessions? If so, what details about these places specifically trigger you?

- Are there any places that you avoid in fear of being triggered?

- What activities increase your experience of uncertainty?

- Lastly, what live scenarios or situations scare you the most?

To help get you thinking of examples, there are some examples below from the ERP Challenge Lists of Alex, Todd, Simone, and Tanya. Read through those, and then fill out your own list.

Alex's ERP Challenge List

- Visit school.
- Hold a bread knife.
- Hold a sharp knife.
- Watch local news.
- Drive past the gun store.
- Walk past the gun store.
- Watch a documentary about pedophiles.
- Watch movies with physical assault or fighting.
- Greet a student in front of the school before class.
- Talk with a student during lunch.
- Ask a student to meet after class to discuss grades.
- Carry a knife in my pocket.
- Allow myself to feel angry.
- Watch a comedy show about violence.
- Bring up a school shooting casually in conversation.
- Share with my best friend about my OCD.

Todd's ERP Challenge List

- Place books down without realigning them.
- Don't check backpack before leaving for school.
- Go to a friend's house after school before doing homework.
- Don't reread books for homework.
- Shower for less than ten minutes.

- Wash hands for less than three minutes.
- Walk through doorways without repeating.
- Turn on lights only one time.
- Step on every stair on the staircase.
- Pack my back for school without counting items.
- Wash my face only one time in the evening.
- Bounce the ball in basketball only when I am playing.
- Don't check my grades more than once per week.

Simone's ERP Challenge List

- Check prescriptions only the recommended amount of times.
- Leave right when my work shift is over, without checking my station.
- Chat with patients when I am administering their prescription.
- Don't check newspaper obituaries.
- Don't call patients to see what they are doing after work.
- Watch medical shows on television.
- Read newspaper articles about immoral people.
- Say prayers only one time, with no repeating.
- Don't confess thoughts to religious minister.
- Attend a church service without engaging in repetitive prayer.
- Make a joke with church friends.
- Look at images of pills and medication on the internet.
- Hold a handful of pills in my hand.
- Carry a bottle of pain medication in my pocket for a full workday.

Tanya's ERP Challenge List

Sexual Orientation Obsessions

- Spend time with men at work.

- Go and have drinks with coworkers after work.

- Spend time with friends who are heterosexual.

- Look at images of handsome men.

- Watch movies with heterosexual intimacy.

- Read articles or blogs about people who have changed sexual orientation.

- Engage in intimacy with Julie.

- Take Julie away for a weekend getaway.

Relationship Obsessions

- Watch television shows about people who cheated on their partners.

- Say "I love you" to Julie when anxious about the purity of my love.

- Spend time away from Julie when anxious about purity of love.

- Discuss relationships with close friends (instead of avoiding such discussions).

- Look at images of women and men online.

- Read blogs about marriage ceremonies.

- Look at wedding rings online without comparing.

Now create your own ERP Challenge List.

_____

_____

_____

_____

_____

_____

_____

_____

_____

_____

_____

_____

Key Points to Remember

Now that you have created your ERP Challenge List, you are ready to start exposure and response prevention. Congratulations! This ERP Challenge List, as daunting as it may seem, will help you take your life back from the repetitive, exhausting cycle of obsessions, compulsions, and self-criticism. As you move forward, I encourage you to remember my favorite saying of all time.

It is a beautiful day to do hard things!

Throughout the next chapters, you will have many opportunities to practice a wide array of ERP exercises. Todd, Alex, Simone, and Tanya will continue to walk alongside you and guide you with their experiences as you practice facing your fears. Let's go!

CHAPTER 6

Self-Compassionate Exposure and Response Prevention

Now that we have your ERP Challenge List ready to go, let's get to work! From here on in, you will practice disrupting the O-C cycle using what I call self-compassionate exposure and response prevention (SC-ERP). Instead of engaging in compulsive safety behaviors, you will practice purposely having your intrusive thoughts, feelings, images, sensations, and urges while treating yourself with the kindness and respect you deserve every step of the way. Using SC-ERP, you will learn that you can tolerate high levels of anxiety, doubt, and uncertainty and that self-criticism and self-punishment do not have to play a role in your life anymore.

Now, I understand that this might feel incredibly daunting. This is completely normal. Facing your fears is no easy feat. However, one thing I know to be true is that *you are exponentially stronger than you could even know.* One of the coolest things about ERP is that you get to learn just how strong you are, and this experience will possibly be the most empowering experience of your life. I have broken down the practice of SC-ERP into four specific steps. These steps will give you a formula for performing exposure and response prevention in a kind, respectful, and compassionate way. The cycle of OCD thrives on self-criticism and self-punishment, so these steps aim to break this cycle and provide you with coping strategies that are nurturing and effective and that bring you closer to the life you want to live.

Below are the four steps of SC-ERP, with each step explained in detail throughout this chapter. With Todd and Tanya by your side as our case studies for this chapter, you will have an opportunity to begin practicing these steps right away. Let's do this!

The Four Steps of Self-Compassionate ERP

1. Intentionally Connect with Your Compassionate Self

2. Self-Compassionate Exposure and Response Prevention

3. Nurture Your Uncertainty and Discomfort with Self-Compassion

4. Reflect, Celebrate, and Repeat

Consider these steps a tried and true way to ensure that your ERP practices are done in the most self-compassionate way possible. I often tell my patients with OCD to consider these steps a recipe for a delicious compassion sandwich. In a compassion sandwich, the main filling of the sandwich (meat and cheese, a vegetarian chickpea spread, grilled mushrooms, lettuce and tomato—whatever you like) is exposure and response prevention, which is the gold-standard treatment for OCD. Self-compassion is the wholesome bread that holds the scrumptious sandwich together and is what allows us to tend to the *entire* person as they courageously stare their fear in the face. As you prepare for your ERP practice and throughout the practice, you will prioritize your own wellness by tending to your discomfort with kindness and consideration. Finally, step 4 (reflect, celebrate, and repeat) is the cookie you treat yourself with after you've finished your compassion sandwich—never stop celebrating yourself and your efforts!

Lastly, while the four steps were developed to help you work through SC-ERP in a step-by-step fashion, it is important that you understand that these steps are fluid and not set in stone. There will be times where you will need to practice these steps in different orders. This is completely fine, so please don't put pressure on yourself to perform them exactly or perfectly.

Step 1: Connect with Your Compassionate Self

Before starting any ERP exercise, you must first connect with the compassionate self that lives within you. Connecting with your compassionate self involves making a radical commitment to unconditionally supporting yourself as you move through your ERP steps and eradicating all forms of self-criticism as your discomfort rises and falls (which it will). Your compassionate self recognizes that you deserve self-compassion, no matter what intrusive thought, image, feeling, sensation, or urge you experience. Your compassionate self is ready to support you no matter how much anticipatory anxiety or uncertainty you experience or how successful or unsuccessful you are at practicing SC-ERP.

So, let's make a deal! From this moment on (yes, forever), you will do your best to be your most significant source of warmth and support throughout all of your ERP practices. You will be the first responder to your own suffering, practicing kindness and respect instead of self-criticism and self-punishment. This practice will involve the removal of not only the harsh, mean words you say to yourself but also any sarcastic, self-deprecating jokes you make about yourself and your obsessions and compulsions. This commitment includes not judging yourself for how well you are coping or how successful you are at your self-compassionate practices.

Last of all, connecting to your compassionate self involves not being hard on yourself when you are struggling with the practice of self-compassion. Simply put, be self-compassionate about your self-compassion practice. I know it's tricky, but it is 100 percent doable!

Putting Your Skills into Practice

Use the space below to write yourself a letter from your compassionate self. This letter will set the scene for being in a self-compassionate mindset as you move through the upcoming exposure and response prevention practices. Feel free to return to this letter as often as needed as you proceed throughout the following steps. If you prefer, you could use the space below to write a bullet-point list of statements inspired by the self-compassion practices you learned in chapter 3. Your self-compassion practice is a personal one, so I encourage you to experiment to find out what does and does not work for you.

_____

_____

_____

_____

_____

_____

_____

_____

_____

_____

Key Points to Remember

Your Compassionate Self

- is *supportive, kind,* and *warm* and has your *best interests at heart;*

- is *encouraging* as you move through the waves of anxiety, uncertainty, and dread;

- brings a *deep wisdom* that knows you can tolerate difficult times and that you are stronger than you have previously given yourself credit;

- helps you *accept* the things you cannot control (your thoughts, feelings, sensations, images, and urges) while you engage with things you can control (your reaction to these obsessions);

- is *motivating* and *empathetic* while holding you *accountable* in a firm but compassionate way;

- does not criticize you or use a condescending or sarcastic voice;

- is *playful* and interested in laughing, and brings *gentle, kind humor,* even during difficult times;

- is *unconditional* and is committed to supporting you even when you fail; and, finally,

- is *nonjudgmental* when you struggle with self-compassion or ERP.

Step 2: Self-Compassionate Exposure and Response Prevention

Now that you have connected with your compassionate self, you are going to practice exposing yourself to your obsessions.

Exposure: Leaning into Your Obsessions

Using your ERP Challenge List created in chapter 5, *identify one challenge item* you are willing to expose yourself to. You may start by identifying an easier challenge item, or, if you are ready to take your OCD down, you can pick a moderate to difficult exposure challenge. Try not to overthink this. There is no "right" way to start this process. It doesn't really matter what order you do exposures in. The only thing that matters is that you work your way through each item on your ERP Challenge List over time, using self-compassion as your superpower.

Response Prevention: The Reduction or Elimination of Compulsions

A successful exposure must include response prevention. Response prevention—the reduction or elimination of compulsive safety behaviors—helps you learn that you can tolerate high levels of anxiety and uncertainty for long periods of time. To practice response prevention, you will need to be willing to be uncertain, uncomfortable, nonjudgmental, curious, present, and of course, self-compassionate to the suffering you experience instead of engaging in compulsions.

Below are Todd's and Tanya's descriptions of their plans for response prevention. Read through their plans and then answer the prompts below to craft your own.

Todd   Todd's primary goal of ERP was to be able to do his homework without getting consumed with compulsions. For this reason, Todd chose to expose himself to his symmetry obsessions by intentionally placing a book on his desk in a random, asymmetrical way. Todd felt it was an easy starter exposure that would give him some practice with being physically uncomfortable around his school materials without being too overwhelming. Once Todd asymmetrically placed his book, he practiced response prevention by withholding from adjusting it back to a symmetrical position for three minutes. Over time, he worked his way up in three-minute increments until he was able to tolerate not adjusting his book back at all.

Tanya   One of Tanya's primary goals of ERP was to be able to spend quality time with her partner again. For this reason, Tanya chose to ask Julie out for a date night as her starter exposure. Tanya had avoided quality time with Julie for some time, as her sexual orientation obsessions and relationship obsessions bombarded her every time they were alone. Tanya identified that her most difficult compulsion to resist was her need to seek reassurance from her partner during their date, but she knew that committing to not asking for reassurance at all was unrealistic and would only set her up to be self-critical and self-punishing. Tanya decided that asking for reassurance two times during date night was more realistic and would also give her the confidence to try to reduce reassurance-seeking during other activities in her day.

Putting Your Skills into Practice

In the space below, identify one item from your ERP Challenge List you would like to start with.

_____

Now, identify how long you would like to challenge yourself to do this exposure for? Is it an ERP activity that requires you to practice exposure for a period of time? Or is it an ERP challenge that requires only engaging in one action or behavior?

_____

Why are you choosing to do this exposure? How will it help you reach your long-term goals?

_____

_____

Using the space below, list the compulsive safety behaviors you would commonly engage in to decrease your anxiety, uncertainty, or discomfort related to the obsession you are exposing yourself to. You may return to your compulsion list from chapter 5, if needed.

_____

_____

How long can you commit to not engaging in these safety behaviors?

_____

SC-ERP Skills

Now that you know what exposure you will do and what response prevention you plan to practice, let's learn some helpful skills to help you stare your fear right in the eyes. These are skills you can practice while engaging in SC-ERP or anytime throughout your day.

- compassionate accountability

- accept uncertainty

- willingness

- non-judgment

- be present in this moment

COMPASSIONATE ACCOUNTABILITY

As discussed in chapter 2, compassionate accountability is the art of coaching yourself through difficult and challenging times in a kind, committed, and encouraging way and without accommodating your fears. As I am sure you know, the feeling of uncertainty, anxiety, and doubt can be incredibly strong, so it is essential that you respond to your fear quite firmly, as you would respond to a bully on the playground. Compassionate accountability involves letting fear know that you will *not* be allowing it to make your decisions or change your mind.

Tanya   Tanya found it helpful to write letters to her OCD (or by speaking to her OCD as if it was a separate person) when she was planning for a difficult exposure.

> *Dear OCD,*
>
> *I am writing to let you know that you are not the boss of me. I no longer am going to allow you to make my decisions. Today, I am going to ask Julie out for a date, and I am not going to let you talk me out of it. I understand that I cannot stop you from coming, but please know that my focus will be on spending time with Julie. You can talk as much as you like, but my attention will be on her.*
>
> *Warmly,*
>
> *Tanya.*

Putting Your Skills into Practice

In the space below, write your own letter to OCD declaring what exposure you will do and how you plan to manage your obsessions and compulsions using compassionate responsibility.

_____

_____

_____

_____

_____

_____

_____

ACCEPT UNCERTAINTY

Accepting uncertainty is one of the most important goals of exposure and response prevention. While you practice your exposures, aim to accept the presence of uncertainty and discomfort without doing compulsions. I understand that this is incredibly difficult, but being uncertain is the tax on being human. Uncertainty is a part of life, and this exposure will help you to be able to tolerate this specific uncertainty just like you do with the million other uncertainties in your life. Try to remind yourself that the presence of uncertainty does not mean your need to resolve or remove it. Below are some examples of how Todd and Tanya practiced accepting their uncertainty.

Todd   "As I do this exposure, I willingly accept the uncertainty that not engaging in compulsions means that I might not be able to think clearly again, which may or may not impact my basketball career and my life success."

After doing his exposures, Todd practiced not solving any of the "What if" thoughts he was experiencing. Todd found it helpful to respond to each intrusive "What if" thought with, "I am choosing not to know" or "Maybe I will. Maybe I won't."

As each thought rolled in, one after the other, he just calmly responded with, "I am not sure" or "Maybe" or "We will just have to see." Responding in this way helped Todd to stay focused on the end goal, which was to practice intentionally leaning into his fears without engaging in safety-seeking behaviors that removed the uncertainty he felt at that moment.

Tanya   "As I do this exposure, I willingly accept the uncertainty that I may never ever know how I feel about my partner or my sexual orientation."

When Tanya went out on her date with Julie, she was overwhelmed with uncertainty. It felt irresponsible to not resolve and figure out what her thoughts meant. Tanya reported that one of the most compassionate things she can do for herself is to give herself permission to just accept what will be and stop beating herself up for not solving this uncertainty.

Putting Your Skills into Practice

In the space below, complete the following sentence: "As I do this exposure, I willingly accept the uncertainty that …" [Insert what uncertainty you are exposing yourself to.]

_____

_____

KEY POINT TO REMEMBER

Think of your recovery using the metaphor of a maze. On one side of the maze is the start and on the other is the finish, with no clear path of how to get from one side to the other. Recovery for OCD is exactly like a maze. Your job is to follow uncertainty. If you are following uncertainty, you are on the right track. If you try to get certainty by doing a compulsion, you will find yourself at a dead-end, and you will need to turn around and return on the path of the uncertainty. This is the only way to get out of the maze. Just remember, if you are leaning into uncertainty, you are going in the right direction.

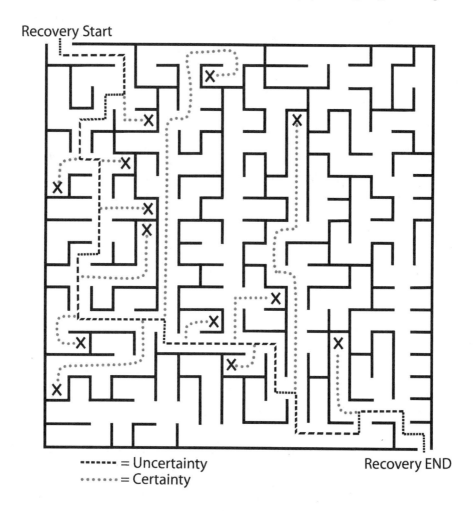

Recovery Start

------- = Uncertainty
·········· = Certainty

Recovery END

WILLINGNESS

When practicing exposures, you are going to experience many moments of physical discomfort. This may be in the form of severe anxiety, panic, disgust, or other sensations that are overwhelmingly uncomfortable. When managing anxiety, whether it is mild anxiety or 10-on-a-scale-of-1-to-10 panic, the golden rule is to *willingly allow it.* You may have already learned that the more you fight discomfort, the worse you will feel.

As you move through an exposure, try to willingly allow your discomfort to rise and fall on its own. If it grows stronger, try not to fight it. Continue to allow whatever you are experiencing, meeting your discomfort with kindness and warmth. If you are concerned that allowing this discomfort or fear will cause you to explode, implode, or even die, return back to your practice of accepting uncertainty. Remember, your amygdala's job is to alert you to every *possible* outcome. But just because you think it, that does not mean it requires an immediate response or, in many cases, a response at all. Gently lean in and learn to respond to your discomfort with compassionate care instead of resistance.

Putting Your Skills into Practice

A great trick to use during exposures is to place your attention on your willingness. Instead of monitoring your anxiety levels, bring your attention to how willing you are to be uncomfortable, on a scale of 1 to 10 (with 1 being not willing at all, and 10 being extremely willing). Here is how Todd practiced this.

Todd   When Todd started his exposure, he rated his willingness to be uncomfortable at a 4 out of 10. Todd and I agreed that he would get much more out of his exposures if he could get his willingness to be uncomfortable to at least a 7 out of 10 (ideally, it would be an 8 or higher). Below are some examples of ways Todd practiced increasing his willingness during exposures:

- Gently breathing steadily as I allow my heart rate to increase or decrease on its own.

- Saying "Bring it on" to the sensations of a full-blown panic attack.

- Softening my stomach muscles as I compassionately leaned into the physical discomfort of stomach distress and cramping.

- Gently unclenching my hands and jaw as I allow the feelings of anxiety to rush through my entire body.

- Allowing my mind to race, allowing all thoughts to arise as they please.

- Allowing the sensation of disgust to be present without clenching my jaw or changing my facial expression to one of repulsion.

Using the same 1-to-10 scale, rate how willing you are to experience this anxiety right now.

1-------2-------3-------4-------5-------6-------7-------8-------9-------10

Now, use the space below to reflect on your willingness to be uncomfortable and how you will address it, as Todd did. Where are you noticing discomfort in your body?

_____

_____

_____

Where in your body are you resisting this discomfort you are experiencing?

_____

_____

_____

How might you increase your willingness to allow this discomfort at this time?

_____

_____

_____

NON-JUDGMENT

After practicing accepting uncertainty and allowing the discomfort, you might start to notice how judgmental you are of what you are experiencing—*This thought is the worst* or *This feeling is awful* or *I am horrible at exposures*. Your reaction to an intrusive thought, image, sensation, feeling, or urge (second arrow) can sometimes determine how painful your experience is. With each negative appraisal, you ensure that you will likely respond in a resistant, compulsive way. Read how Tanya worked through this and try it yourself.

Tanya   Tanya worked very hard in therapy to replace negative judgment with more objective, nonjudgmental responses. When Tanya did her exposure, she practiced saying, "I am observing thoughts about infidelity right now" (nonjudgmental approach) instead of "I am a horrible person for thinking about cheating. What is wrong with me?" (highly judgmental).

Remember, for as long as you are alive, you will have all kinds of thoughts, feelings, sensations, images, and urges. Your job is to practice not infusing them with stories of judgment and negativity.

Putting Your Skills into Practice

As you do your exposure, use the space below to list some of the judgments you place on your thoughts, feelings, sensations, urges, and on you as a whole.

_____

_____

How do you feel when you judge them harshly?

_____

_____

Using Tanya's example, identify your judgmental statements and then try to restructure them to a nonjudgmental statement. I encourage you to use spare paper if you have many judgmental statements and comments about yourself and your experience of anxiety, uncertainty, and discomfort.

_____

_____

_____

_____

BE PRESENT IN THIS MOMENT

While you engage in your exposure, or even before you engage in your exposure, you will likely experience some hypervigilance and anticipatory anxiety about whether your fear will come true or not. As you lean into your fear, you will naturally want to focus on all possible bad outcomes that may or may not occur in the future. You might also notice that once you have done the exposure, your mind will want to go back into the past and review what happened, how you felt, and why you felt that way. These behaviors are considered mental compulsions. As you practice doing your exposure, try to place your attention only on *this* present moment. What are you aware of right now? Where are you? What is happening around you right now? This act of inquiring is what connects us to this present moment. Instead of focusing on what *will* happen or what *did* happen, focus on what *is* happening in this moment.

Tanya   While on her date, Tanya practiced being present by connecting with her five senses. Tanya observed the sounds of her partner's voice and the sounds at the restaurant, the smell of the food, what colors she could see, and what it felt like for the gravity to pull her down toward the earth's surface. As Tanya engaged in her exposure, she had many intrusive thoughts and sexual images that raised her anxiety and uncertainty. Each and every time (and yes, there were many), Tanya practiced not judging her thoughts or images and then practiced compassionately bringing her attention back to the present.

Putting Your Skills into Practice

Using the space below, document what you notice is happening right now as you do your SC-ERP. What do you see, hear, smell, taste, feel? What shapes and colors do you see? What does the air feel like against your skin?

_____

_____

_____

_____

What is getting in the way of you being present during your SC-ERP challenge?

_____

_____

_____

_____

Don't Forget—It Is a Beautiful Day to Do Hard Things!

SOMETIMES, LIFE IS AN EXPOSURE!

You may find that there are many times during the day when you will not need to seek out exposures, as life, in general, creates its own impromptu exposures (lucky you!). Maybe a family member does something that triggers your obsessions, or you see a billboard on the side of the highway or an ad on television that triggers an intrusive thought. In these cases, use it as an opportunity to practice response prevention. Your objective is to embrace the uncertainty, anxiety, and discomfort that arises and then to put as much energy as you can into not engaging in compulsions. These unplanned exposures are just as important as the ones you plan and purposely execute. Again, you may choose to go all out with response prevention and withhold all compulsions, or you may choose to set a time limit (similar to what Tanya did) for how long you plan to willingly tolerate your discomfort without engaging in compulsions.

Something to Consider: Be Prepared for Your Thoughts to Get Loud!

You may notice that during your SC-ERP practices, the frequency and volume of your intrusive thoughts often get *really loud*. The content of these intrusive thoughts aren't more important than your regular obsessions. In fact, they are often the exact same thoughts you have day in and day out. One difference is that they turn your "What if" thoughts into even more catastrophized statements. They are louder, meaner, and demand that you act compulsively *right now!* These intrusive thoughts come in all shapes and sizes, depending on your subtype, but some common examples include:

- "This exposure will cause something *really* bad to happen!"

- "You are an irresponsible fool if you do this exposure!"

- "Stop! Your compulsions prevent the bad things from happening!"

- "But this is the one time that this is *real*!"

- "This is proof that you are a horrible person!"

- "This exposure will make you snap and lose control!"

- "But what if this is not OCD?"

These intrusive thoughts have one main goal: to get you to engage back in compulsions. As you move through your ERP Challenge List, do your best to become aware of these catastrophized thoughts and how they lure you into engaging in safety-seeking compulsions. Just as with any obsession, your goal is to practice leaning into your fear and tenderly holding space for the uncertainty, fear, and discomfort that arises within you. You can do this! It is just a matter of learning how to play OCD's game!

Step 3: Nurture with Self-Compassion

In step 3, you will create a safe place for whatever discomfort or suffering you are experiencing. You might be feeling anxiety, panic, uncertainty, doubt, anger, shame, guilt, overwhelm, frustration, exhaustion, grief, or whatever else is left over after doing ERP. This step is the catch-all for everything you are feeling. If you feel angry, be kind to yourself. If you feel completely out of control, be kind to yourself. If you think you are going to have a massive panic attack, be kind to yourself. If you struggled with response prevention, be kind to yourself. If you have no anxiety at all—and this concerns you— be kind to yourself.

The step of nurturing is treating yourself with the same compassion and care you would give another person who was going through a similar situation. You may want to go back and ask yourself how you would treat a loved one if they were experiencing the same degree of anxiety, panic, or distress. You can rely on any of the tools discussed in this workbook in this step, and I encourage you to play around with different tools to see what works and what doesn't work. There will be days when one of the self-compassion tools you used is not as helpful or may not resonate as much as it had previously. That is totally okay. Just listen to your body and continue to inquire into what it needs during this difficult time. Try to remember that compulsions only provide temporary relief and only push you back into the cycle of obsessions and compulsions. However, self-compassion and nurturing bring with them long-term, unconditional care during even the worst moment of anxiety and fear.

Putting Your Skills into Practice

In the space below, reflect on what it is that you need during this present moment. What is it that you need to hear right now?

_____

_____

_____

_____

Are there any self-compassion practices that you feel will assist you at this time?

_____

_____

_____

_____

Step 4: Reflect, Celebrate, and Repeat!

Well done for getting to step 4! This step is where you take stock of what went well and what did not go so well. This step can provide you many insights about how you handle yourself in difficult and distressing times. Reflecting your SC-ERP progress can help you to learn more about your specific cycle of obsessions and compulsions and help you to identify specific points where you need to intervene with a particular tool or practice. While reflecting your experience with self-compassionate ERP, be very mindful of your critical voice stepping in and taking over. Try to reflect on your successes and challenges in a kind and encouraging way. Remember, self-compassionate ERP is a work in progress, so it is entirely okay if you made lots of mistakes and identify lots of roadblocks. With time and practice, you will learn these skills, and they will become a part of your daily life.

Todd   During Todd's reflection, Todd practiced using his kind coach voice. Todd really resonated with the concept of being his own kind coach, as he had lots of previous experience with both the mean and kind coaches, and this distinction helped him to navigate which voice he needed to use. As Todd reflected on his progress, he identified several areas where he could improve. Todd noticed that when doing his exposures, he struggled to tolerate his discomfort. While he was successful at not realigning the book, he did catch himself engaging in other compulsions, specifically mental rumination. Todd identified that he might succeed more in future ERP if he became more aware of this and practiced his mindfulness and self-compassion skills more during response prevention. Todd knew that the complete extinction of mental rumination was unlikely, so for future ERP, he made the compassionate and realistic goal of not engaging in mental rumination for approximately three to five minutes and then worked his way up to more extended periods from there.

Reflection

Using the space below, reflect on the questions provided.

Did you engage in any self-criticism during these steps? If so, how did you handle yourself once you realized this? What self-compassion tools will you try next time you practice ERP?

_____

_____

_____

_____

Was the exposure challenging enough? What can you do in the future to make it a little harder?

_____

_____

_____

_____

How willing were you to do the exposure? What could you do in the future to increase your willingness to be uncomfortable?

_____

_____

_____

_____

What tools do you need to focus on next time you practice facing your fears?

_____

_____

_____

_____

What thoughts, feelings, sensations, urges, and images got in the way of your response prevention? If you were not successful, what self-compassion skills can you use to hold yourself more accountable next time?

_____

_____

_____

_____

_____

Now that you have reflected on your progress, it is time to *celebrate*! Get up and do a happy dance, even if your anxiety is through the roof. Always be sure to celebrate every single time you attempted to face your fears, even if it didn't go well. ERP is one of the hardest things you will ever do in your lifetime, so do not forget to give yourself a mental high-five, call a friend to share how hard you tried, or do something nice for yourself to show recognition of this brave and courageous work you are doing. Below is Tanya's list of ways to celebrate.

Tanya's Celebratory List

Say out loud: "I am proud of you, Tanya!"

Say out loud: "You did a hard thing. Well done!"

Say out loud: "I am a badass!"

Take a warm bath.

Dance or jump up and down with pride.

Tell a friend about my accomplishment.

Share my success in a private online OCD group.

Putting Your Skills into Practice

In the space below, list three to five things you could say to yourself or do to celebrate your attempts at self-compassionate ERP.

_____

_____

_____

_____

_____

Repeat, Repeat, Repeat!

Now that you have successfully worked through all of the steps of self-compassionate ERP, your job is to *repeat* these steps over and over until you complete all of the items on your ERP Challenge List without doing compulsions. Now, I understand that this might seem like the most colossal concept ever, so please remember to give yourself permission to take baby steps and work through these steps using realistic and compassionate goals.

As you work through your ERP Challenge List, try to find as many opportunities to practice self-compassionate ERP in as many different situations as possible. Tanya and Todd share some examples on the next page.

Tanya   One of the exposures on Tanya's ERP Challenge List was to go out for lunch with a colleague at work without mentally reviewing her sexual orientation or asking for reassurance. Tanya did her best to arrange luncheon meetings with as many different people as possible, instead of having lunch with the same person repeatedly for her exposure. This allowed Tanya to practice managing various obsessions and compulsions that arose in each different situation.

Todd   Todd chose to first start exposures by placing his book on his desk asymmetrically. He then added items such as his toothbrush, clothing drawers, and curtains, just to name a few. Then Todd practiced asymmetrically placing these items in every room in his house and then moved on to practice this same ERP challenge at school, at his grandmother's home, and then at friends' houses. The ultimate exposure was to practice placing items asymmetrically at his basketball court and in the classroom during academic tests. Todd also practiced allowing or creating events that induced the "not right" feeling as much as he could throughout the day in as many different contexts as possible.

How Much Self-Compassionate ERP Should I Be Aiming For?

As a guide, try to aim for approximately forty-five to ninety minutes of self-compassionate ERP per day. You can use this time to complete any of the exposures from your ERP Challenge List, or you can use this time to practice any of the self-compassionate ERP practices from chapters 7 to 10.

You can schedule your self-compassionate ERP in blocks, or you can find ways to infuse your exposures and response prevention into your everyday routine. Either way is excellent, as long as you give yourself ample time to practice leaning into your fears and using the tools you have learned from this chapter.

Reflection

Realistically, when are the best times for you to schedule your self-compassionate ERP? All at once? Or broken into smaller time slots? Be as specific as you can. Once you have identified some good times, put them into your calendar.

_____

_____

Now that you have completed one self-compassionate ERP exercise, list as many ways as possible to practice this exposure in different settings.

_____

_____

_____

_____

_____

_____

The rest of the workbook will provide you with many opportunities to practice the four steps of self-compassionate ERP. In the following chapters, you will learn how to apply these steps to different types of exposures, such as imaginal scripts, flooding exposures, interoceptive exposures, and exposure games. To ensure that you include each step, I have created the worksheet below. You may use this as a cheat sheet to prepare for upcoming exposures, or you can use it in real time as you practice facing your obsessions using your ERP Challenge List. You may download a PDF of this worksheet from this book's website (http://www.newharbinger.com/47766).

My Self-Compassionate ERP Plan

Step 1: Connect with Your Compassionate Self (How can you support and encourage yourself as you move into your exposure?)

_____

_____

_____

Step 2: Self-Compassionate Exposure and Response Prevention

Exposure (Pick one from your ERP Challenge List)

_____

_____

Response Prevention (What compulsions do you need to resist engaging in?)

_____

_____

_____

Step 3: Nurture Your Anxiety, Uncertainty, and Discomfort (What self-compassion practices will you use as you nurture your anxiety, uncertainty, and discomfort?)

_____

_____

_____

Step 4: Reflect, Celebrate, and Repeat (What went well? What do you need to work on? How can you make this exposure more challenging in the future?)

_____

_____

_____

CHAPTER 7

Self-Compassionate Flooding Exposures

When my daughter was a young toddler, she exercised her curiosity by turning on the faucet to the bathroom sink and watched and waited until the sink overflowed. Water quickly flooded over the entire floor, moving so quickly that it also flooded the carpet of the room next door. Metaphorically, this is the process of doing flooding exposures.

As my daughter did, flooding exposures are all about metaphorically "turning on the faucet" to your intrusive thoughts and allowing your obsessions to overflow to all the spaces inside and around you.

In this chapter, you will identify the specific intrusive thoughts that trigger you and then practice repeating them over and over (exposure using flooding) while practicing embracing your anxiety and uncertainty instead of doing compulsions (response prevention). Simone will be your case study for this chapter and will walk alongside you as you use all four steps of self-compassionate ERP. Using a gradual exposure format, you will start with a moderately easy flooding exposure and work your way up to flooding your most difficult fears.

Step 1: Connect with Your Compassionate Self

Take a moment before each flooding exercise to check in with your compassionate self.

Putting Your Skills into Practice

What would your compassionate self say to you right now? What do you need right now to help support, nurture, and motivate yourself to engage in the upcoming flooding exposures?

_____

_____

_____

_____

_____

Using the space below, reflect on your experience of connecting to your compassionate self. Are you committed to continuing your self-compassion practices throughout your upcoming ERP? Remember, even the _intention_ to be self-compassionate is moving you in the right direction.

_____

_____

_____

_____

_____

Step 2: Self-Compassionate Exposure and Response Prevention

There are three different levels of flooding exposures in this chapter, starting with the easiest and progressing to the most difficult exposures. The pace in which you perform these flooding exposures is entirely up to you. You may choose to slowly work your way through the different flooding exposures, one at a time, or you may choose to do all of the flooding exercises in this chapter in one swoop. Either way, please don't forget the importance of self-compassionate response prevention during each flooding exercise.

Putting Your Skills into Practice

Flooding Exposures: Write Your Obsession Down!

First, identify one word that causes a low-to-moderate degree of anxiety or uncertainty. Using the space below, write the word at least twenty times—slowly and clearly. Try to really let the word permeate your experience, without rushing, scribbling, or modifying the word to make it less uncomfortable. As you write, look at the word and allow whatever discomfort you feel to rise and fall. Simone gives you an example.

Simone: "Medication Medication"

_____

_____

_____

Once you have completed this flooding exposure, use the space below to repeat the writing exposure using a moderately difficult word.

Simone: "Sin Sin Sin Sin Sin Sin Sin Sin Sin Sin Sin Sin Sin Sin Sin Sin Sin Sin Sin Sin Sin Sin Sin Sin Sin Sin Sin Sin Sin Sin Sin Sin Sin Sin Sin Sin"

_____

_____

_____

Once you have completed this flooding exposure, use the space below to repeat the writing exposure using your most challenging, triggering word.

Simone: "Sinner Sinner"

_____

_____

_____

Flooding Exposures: Say Your Obsessions Out Loud!

You will now practice repetitively saying your specific obsession out loud. Using the words from the previous flooding exercises, repeat each word—starting with the easiest word and working your way up to the most challenging word—aloud, slowly, and clearly for approximately thirty seconds. It is natural to want to rush through this process, but do your best to intentionally say the words, allowing your experience of anxiety and uncertainty as you say the words aloud. If you get distracted by your obsessions, start thinking about something else, or if you begin engaging in a compulsive safety-seeking behavior, try not to become critical of yourself. This is to be expected. If your mind goes off track, gently bring your attention back to the flooding exposure.

Flooding Exposures: Record Your Obsessions and Listen Back!

Once you have practiced saying the thought out loud, use a smartphone or other audio device to record yourself saying your specific obsession aloud for a particular amount of time. I encourage all of my clients to do this for a minimum of three minutes, but I have found that five to six minutes is usually best, which allows enough time to say the word approximately one hundred times. Consider this a real accomplishment! Bravo! Once you have recorded yourself flooding, listen back to the recording every day as many times as possible. Think of these exposures like mental pushups. The more you do, the stronger you get!

Flooding Exposures: Lean into Your Obsession a Little More!

Okay, now we turn that faucet on a little more, and we move up to flooding with full sentences. In the space below, you will create three sentences related to your specific obsession. Again, Simone helps out with her own examples.

In the space below, write a moderately easy sentence about your specific obsession coming true. Try to write in the present tense and be as courageous as you can.

Simone: "I mix up the medication, and my patient gets sick."

_____

_____

_____

Now, using the space below, write a moderately difficult sentence about your feared consequence.

Simone: "I mix up the medication, and my patient gets sick and dies."

_____

_____

_____

Using the space below, now write your *most difficult* sentence. The most difficult sentence should involve more details and specifics about your fear coming true.

Simone: "I am a sinner. I purposely mix up the medication, and my patient dies an excruciating death."

_____

_____

_____

Once you have written out these sentences, practice saying them out loud, twenty times for each one, as you did in the previous exercise, and then move on to recording yourself saying the sentences aloud for three to six minutes each. Try to really imagine yourself in these situations and let your mind go, allowing any additional thoughts, feelings, sensations, and urges to arise.

Once you have completed all of the flooding exposures in this chapter, work your way up to flooding for five or even fifteen minutes per day. There is no limit to how much you engage in flooding exposures. You can listen back to your flooding recordings or flood in your head while you take the train to work, wash the dishes, take a shower, or while doing any other daily activity. You will also find it incredibly beneficial to practice your flooding exposures *while* you do your exposures from your ERP Challenge List. Flooding exposures are particularly effective when doing exposures to the people, events, and places you have previously avoided.

Response Prevention

Using the space below, reflect on your practice of response prevention. Before, during, and after engaging in your flooding exposures, were there any compulsions you felt compelled to perform? If so, which compulsions? Simone gives an example to guide you.

Simone: "Since doing my flooding exposure, I really want to go back to the medication vault and check which medication I actually administered my patient. Even though I know this would relieve my anxiety and uncertainty, I am committed to not doing this compulsion."

_____

_____

_____

_____

What tools and practices can you use to help you resist the urge to engage in safety-seeking compulsions?

Simone: "I am going to practice tolerating the uncertainty and re-engage in what it is that I was doing before I did my exposure. I am going to go back to responding to emails and preparing my lunch."

_____

_____

_____

_____

Step 3: Nurture Anxiety, Uncertainty, and Doubt

It is likely that these exposures brought on a large degree of anxiety, uncertainty, or maybe a strong wave of multiple emotions. If this is the case, try not to resist what you are experiencing. Take this time to really make space and compassionately tend to the discomfort and suffering you are currently facing. Simone gives an example of how she handled it.

Putting Your Skills into Practice

Using the space below, check in with yourself and notice if you are experiencing any discomfort in your body right now. If so, where do you notice this discomfort?

Simone: "It is really hard not to use unkind words at this time. I feel a great deal of judgment toward myself for the thoughts I am having and the guilt I feel. As I move on to checking my emails and preparing my lunch, I will practice compassionate breathing and compassionate touch. I know that the most badass thing I can do right now is to sit tight in my discomfort and treat myself kindly. So I am going to try my best."

_____

_____

_____

What can you do right now to help support yourself as you gently allow the anxiety, uncertainty, and discomfort you feel? Is there a self-compassion practice that might help you stay tender as you willingly experience discomfort? If so, take as much time as you need to practice this exercise now.

_____

_____

_____

_____

Step 4: Reflect, Celebrate, and Repeat

Reflect on your experience in the following exercise.

Reflection

How willing were you to experience discomfort, anxiety, and uncertainty related to this thought? (1 being little willingness and 10 being very willing)

1-------2-------3-------4-------5-------6-------7-------8-------9-------10

How successful were you at not judging yourself negatively or being self-critical? (1 being "I was not self-judgmental at all" and 10 being "I engaged in a lot of self-judgment and self-criticism.")

1-------2-------3-------4-------5-------6-------7-------8-------9-------10

How successful was I at practicing response prevention? How might I set myself up for success with this in the future?

Simone: "I did mostly really well, I think. However, I did struggle with not engaging with mental compulsions, trying to solve if I liked the words I was flooding."

_____

_____

_____

_____

What could you do to create a more compassionate experience as you practice flooding exposures?

Simone: "I could give myself radical permission to feel whatever it is that I am feeling, without judging myself as good or bad."

_____

_____

_____

How could you increase your willingness to being uncertain and uncomfortable? Is there a compassionate phrase or statement that empowers and motivates you? What tools could you practice as you move forward with these exposures?

Simone: "Bring on the anxiety, baby! It's a beautiful day to do hard things!"

_____

_____

_____

In the future, is there a way to make these flooding exposures more difficult? Is there a location or a person you could expose yourself to while you practice these flooding exposures? How can you challenge yourself in these exposures?

Simone: "I can do these flooding exercises while I am at work, dispensing medication. I could also listen to my flooding exposure recordings over and over at night when I feel the need to engage in mentally reviewing what I did and did not do at work that day."

_____

_____

_____

Something to Look Out For

Todd identified during his symptom assessment that one of the biggest reasons he performed symmetry and "just right" compulsions was to neutralize his fear of becoming unsuccessful. His obsession was that if he did not align things in a "just right way," his future success would be dismal. Todd decided that the most effective flooding sentence he could use would be "I become unsuccessful." Todd reported that this exposure had the opposite effect on him than he expected and that he felt strangely reassured after he said his flooding sentences aloud. When I inquired about this, Todd reported that flooding "I become unsuccessful" sounded ridiculous, and he enjoyed the small moments of relief these exposures provided him. Todd reported he was practicing these flooding exposures many, many times per day. I explained to Todd that it sounded like he was using flooding as a _compulsion_ instead of an _exposure_. This was quite confusing for Todd at first, but when he consulted with his _why_, he realized he was using flooding to _remove_ anxiety and uncertainty instead of leaning into anxiety and uncertainty. Todd spent some time troubleshooting this and found that flooding was only effective at increasing his anxiety and uncertainty when he combined it with physically misaligning an object such as a book or a trophy.

CHAPTER 8

Self-Compassionate Imaginal Exposures

Congratulations on all of your hard work so far! Bravo! You should be so proud of yourself for honoring your mental health and taking steps to take back your life from OCD.

In this chapter, you will practice staring your fear *right in the face*, practicing imaginal exposures. Imaginal exposures, also called "scripting," involve simulating your obsessions by writing detailed stories about your fear coming true. Scripting gives you the opportunity to expose yourself to the fine details of your most anxiety-inducing fears so you can then practice tolerating the anxiety, uncertainty, and doubt that arise. Imaginal scripts are also excellent ways to practice self-compassionate ERP when logistics, time, and resources get in the way. Once you have written and read your scripts, you can use them as an opportunity to strengthen your response-prevention skills and your mindfulness and self-compassion practices.

In this chapter, with Tanya's, Simone's, and Todd's guidance, you will learn how to write three different types of imaginal exposures. All three scripts have their own specific objective and are an incredibly important part of your ERP plan.

The three types of imaginal scripts we will be using are:

- worst-case-scenario scripts

- uncertainty scripts

- acceptance scripts

SC-ERP Using Worst-Case-Scenario Scripts

Worst-case-scenario scripts are used to purposely induce the most catastrophic, anxiety-provoking intrusive thoughts related to your obsession, so that you can practice tolerating the discomfort, anxiety, and uncertainty, and then engage in successful response prevention.

Step 1: Connect with Your Compassionate Self

The very idea of performing these scripts can be overwhelming and anxiety provoking. It is common to have high levels of anticipatory anxiety combined with strong emotions such as shame, guilt, and disgust. For this reason, you must tenderly nurture these emotions using your self-compassion practices.

Putting Your Skills into Practice

Using the space below, reflect on what emotions arise in anticipation of this exercise. How do you habitually respond to these feelings?

_____

_____

_____

_____

What intrusive thoughts are you observing as you prepare for these upcoming exposures? Are you judging them as "good" or "bad"?

_____

_____

_____

What would you like your compassionate self to say to you as you move into this exposure?

_____

_____

_____

_____

Step 2: Self-Compassionate ERP

Using your list of obsessions created in chapter 5, pick one moderately easy obsession. Now, using the worst-case-scenario script template below, create a story about this obsession coming true. Your goal is to introduce as many small details as you can to help you visualize and embrace this narrative.

Try to keep in mind that when it comes to writing scripts, there is *no topic* that is off-limits. Make it your goal to write a script that is equally as graphic as the intrusive thoughts that present themselves in your mind each day. The juicier the obsession, the more in detail you can go into your scripts.

Putting Your Skills into Practice

Using the prompts provided below, first write a basic script based on the obsession you picked for this exposure. Tanya will walk alongside you as you write your worst-case-scenario script.

Exposure: Basic Script Template

Title: [Insert the obsession you are targeting.]

Tanya: "The day I realize I am a heterosexual."

_____

"I am ..." [Insert where your fear occurs here.]

Tanya: "I am at work."

_____

"I am ..." [Insert who you are with and what you are doing before your fear occurred here.]

Tanya: "I see Samuel, a male coworker, in the lunchroom."

_____

_____

In the section below, write a few sentences about your obsession coming true. These sentences should be in the present tense and always be written in the first person.

Tanya: "I am overwhelmed with attraction and arousal for Samuel. I realize I am a heterosexual. I have sex with Samuel on the lunchroom table. I have to tell Julie that I cheated on her."

_____

_____

_____

_____

"I spend the rest of my life ..." [Insert what the consequences of your obsessions would be, if they came true.]

Tanya: "I spend the rest of my life alone and unhappy. I never find anyone else like Julie, and I am miserable forever."

_____

_____

_____

Great work! Now, you will practice writing a more advanced script using the template provided below. In this exercise, you work toward writing scripts that are up to a full page long. The goal is to include as much detail as possible in your scripts. However, it is important to understand that the length really doesn't matter. What matters is that you practice allowing your intrusive thoughts and images of the feared situation, then willingly tolerate the anxiety, uncertainty, and discomfort they induce.

Exposure: Advanced Script Template

"I am ..." [Insert where your fear occurs here. Include details about this location such as what you see, hear, smell, and so forth.]

Tanya: "I am at work, and I see a colleague go into the lunchroom."

_____

_____

_____

"I am ..." [Insert specific details about what you are doing before your feared outcome occurred here.]

Tanya: "I walk in, and I see Samuel standing at the sink. He is wearing tight business pants, and I can see the outline of his pants around his buttocks and genital area."

_____

_____

_____

_____

In the section below, write one or two paragraphs about your obsession coming true or the uncertainty of your obsession. The more detailed and explicit, the better.

Tanya: "I am overwhelmed with arousal and desire to kiss him. I do everything I can to stop myself, but the desire and arousal are too strong, and I find an excuse to go into the lunchroom. I push the man up against the wall and start kissing him. I am aroused more than I have ever been in my entire life. We have sex right on the lunch counter, and I'm shocked at how pleasurable it was. As I leave the lunchroom, I realize that I am not homosexual. I am a heterosexual who is attracted to men. I have to go home and tell Julie that I disrespected and dishonored her by cheating on her with a man. Julie is devastated. She and I separate, and I live my life alone, still not having complete certainty on whether I am gay or straight. Julie goes off and marries somebody else and has a happier life."

_____

_____

_____

_____

_____

_____

_____

"I spend the rest of my life ..." [Insert the irreversible consequences of your obsessions, if they came true.]

Tanya: "I spend the rest of my life alone, and everyone hates me for what I have done."

_____

_____

_____

_____

RESPONSE PREVENTION

As you practice reading your worst-case-scenario script, you will likely have some pretty strong emotions arise, and you will notice strong urges to engage in compulsions in order to make the discomfort subside. Try to use this as a golden opportunity to hold space for those emotions while maintaining a respectful and compassionate environment for yourself.

Putting Your Skills into Practice

Use the journal prompts below to help you wade through these moments of discomfort.

On a scale of 1 to 10 (with 1 being not willing at all and 10 being very willing), how willing were you to immerse yourself in your worst-case-scenario script?

1-------2-------3-------4-------5-------6-------7-------8-------9-------10

Were there any additional thoughts, feelings, images, sensations, and urges that arose as you read these scripts?

_____

_____

_____

Are there any compulsions you feel compelled to engage in? If so, what behaviors or activities can you do instead of engaging in these compulsive acts?

_____

_____

_____

_____

Step 3: Nurture Anxiety, Uncertainty, and Doubt

As you move through this exposure and as you practice response prevention, your goal is to meet your discomfort in a kind and compassionate way.

Putting Your Skills into Practice

Are you noticing any self-criticism or self-judgment right now? If so, how does this make you feel?

_____

_____

_____

How might you practice meeting your discomfort, uncertainty, or anxiety with self-compassion instead of using self-criticism or self-judgment?

_____

_____

_____

If you connect with your compassionate self, what do you need to hear right now that might help you move forward with response prevention in a nonjudgmental way?

_____

_____

_____

Step 4: Reflect, Celebrate, and Repeat

In the space below, reflect on your experience with practicing worst-case-scenario scripts, and use the prompts below to help you review your progress, celebrate your attempts, and plan for future self-compassionate ERP.

Reflection

Reflect

On a scale of 1 to 10 (with 1 being not judgmental at all and 10 being highly judgmental and self-critical), how successful were you at not judging yourself negatively or being self-critical during this activity?

1-------2-------3-------4-------5-------6-------7-------8-------9-------10

Did you engage in any compulsive behaviors during this scripting exercise? If so, which compulsions did you engage in?

_____

What got in the way of your willingness to be uncertain and uncomfortable during this scripting exercise? What could you do to increase your willingness to be uncomfortable instead of engaging in compulsive behaviors?

_____

_____

_____

_____

What could you do before, during, and after these scripting exercises to create a more compassionate experience as you practice scripting exposures?

_____

_____

_____

Celebrate

How can you celebrate your success with this exposure? What could you say to motivate, support, and encourage yourself to keep going with SC-ERP?

_____

_____

_____

Repeat, Repeat, Repeat!

What could you do to make this scripting exposure a little more challenging for next time?

_____

_____

_____

How often can you commit to doing these exposures?

_____

How will you incorporate them into your everyday routine?

_____

Now that you have written your scripts, I encourage you to read them in all of the places you are afraid your fear will come true. If this is not possible, or if you want to work your way up to reading it at your feared location, feel free to read it wherever it is convenient. Start with reading it just once, slowly and intentionally, trying to imagine it happening. From there, move your way up to reading it ten to twenty times per day. While this might seem like a lot, please remember that SC-ERP requires a lot of practice. Aim to include worst-case-scenario scripts into your forty-five to ninety minutes of SC-ERP per day.

Another option is to record yourself slowly reading your scripts using a recording app or smartphone and listen to it over and over on your way to work, as you walk the dogs, or during any activity you choose. This can be especially helpful if you are struggling to find time in your schedule to do your exposures. As you repeat these scripts, try to focus on immersing yourself in the imagery of the story and its small details.

Self-Compassionate ERP Using Uncertainty Scripts

Uncertainty scripts might seem similar to worst-case-scenario scripts, but they serve a different fundamental purpose when it comes to exposure and response prevention. Instead of writing about your worst fear coming true, uncertainty scripts set out to expose you to the uncertainty related to your worst fear coming true. Many people with OCD report that the experience of having uncertainty around a particular event happening is equally, if not more, concerning than imagining the worst-case-scenario. For this reason, you are going to practice exposing yourself directly to the uncertainty and give yourself another opportunity to tolerate it while practicing response prevention and self-compassion.

Step 1: Connect with Your Compassionate Self

Use the space below to reflect on your experience with uncertainty. This will involve gently acknowledging the suffering that comes with experiencing uncertainty. Try to do your best to meet your resistance and aversion to uncertainty by connecting with the compassionate self that lives within you.

Putting Your Skills into Practice

What emotions, sensations, or thoughts arise when you think about uncertainty?

_____

_____

_____

Is there a place in your body that is particularly resistant right now? If so, what can you do to meet that discomfort compassionately and mindfully?

_____

_____

_____

What compassionate act can you practice before leaning into uncertainty? Is there a self-compassion practice that could help you nurture your discomfort right now instead of trying to make it go away?

_____

_____

_____

Step 2: Self-Compassionate ERP

Using your list of obsessions created in chapter 5, identify the obsession that causes you the most uncertainty. An easy way to do this is by asking yourself, "What obsession do I spend the most time trying to solve or find the answer to?" Once you have it, use the template below to create your own uncertainty script. The goal of your uncertainty script is to sit in the experience of not knowing and commit to being uncertain about what will happen in your future. Once again, try your hardest to describe the experience of being uncertain about your obsession. Simone's uncertainty scripts are shown after the instruction for your reference.

Putting Your Skills into Practice

Exposure: Uncertainty Script Template

I am ... [Describe a situation in which you will never find certainty about your fear. Where are you? What are you doing? Who are you with?]

Simone: "I'm at work, and I am filling prescriptions behind the pharmacy counter. I perform the mandatory check that the medication and prescription are the same. I dispense the medication to the patient, and the patient pays the pharmacy and leaves. The next day I return to work, and one of the pharmacy assistants tells us that one of our patients has died. No one knows the cause of death, and everyone in the pharmacy is shocked, because the patient was healthy and had just been in yesterday."

_____

_____

_____

_____

_____

_____

"I realize that I will never know ..." [Insert the obsessions you are uncertain about.]

Simone: "I realize that I will never know exactly why they died."

_____

_____

"Because of this uncertainty, I spend the rest of my life ..." [Insert the consequences of not having certainty in your life.]

Simone: "Because of this uncertainty, I spend the rest of my life not knowing whether I am responsible for this person's death. I will never know if it was because of an error I made. I attend the funeral of this patient, and I see how heartbroken the family is. I live with this uncertainty for the rest of my life."

_____

_____

_____

_____

Once you have written your uncertainty script, read it aloud, slowly and clearly. Mindfully and self-compassionately allow the images, thoughts, and experience or uncertainty that arises.

RESPONSE PREVENTION

Once you have written and read your uncertainty script, you will now lean in and make space for the uncertainty and anxiety you feel. Again, try to resist the urge to engage in safety-seeking compulsions. Use the prompts below to help you practice self-compassionate response prevention.

Putting Your Skills into Practice

Does the experience of uncertainty increase your urge to perform any specific compulsions? If so, which ones?

_____

_____

_____

_____

_____

_____

On a scale of 1 to 10 (with 1 being not willing at all and 10 being very willing), how willing are you to allow uncertainty at this moment without engaging in compulsions?

1-------2-------3-------4-------5-------6-------7-------8-------9-------10

Step 3: Nurture Anxiety, Uncertainty, and Doubt

Now that you have written your uncertainty script and are practicing response prevention, use the prompts below to help you nurture the discomfort that arises.

Putting Your Skills into Practice

As you move through this SC-ERP exercise, what emotional suffering needs tending to? How might you acknowledge your discomfort without judging it, pushing it away, or trying to solve it?

_____

_____

_____

_____

What self-compassion practices could support you as you allow your anxiety and uncertainty to rise and fall?

_____

_____

How can you make space for the uncertainty without criticizing yourself, catastrophizing your future, or resisting it?

_____

_____

_____

Step 4: Reflect, Celebrate, and Repeat

Using the prompts below, reflect on your experience with uncertainty scripts.

Reflection

Reflect

On a scale of 1 to 10 (with 1 being not judgmental at all and 10 being highly judgmental and self-critical), how successful were you at not judging yourself negatively or being self-critical during this activity?

1-------2-------3-------4-------5-------6-------7-------8-------9-------10

Did you engage in any compulsive behaviors during this exposure? If so, which compulsions did you engage in?

_____

_____

What got in the way of your willingness to be uncertain? What could you do to increase your willingness to be uncomfortable to help you resist engaging in compulsive behaviors?

_____

_____

_____

What could you do before, during, and after these exposures to create a more compassionate experience as you practice being aware of uncertainty?

_____

_____

_____

Celebrate

How can you celebrate your successes with this exposure? Is there someone safe and supportive you can share this with? What could you say to yourself or do for yourself to encourage and motivate you to keep going?

_____

_____

_____

Repeat, Repeat, Repeat!

What could you do next time to make this script a little more challenging?

_____

_____

_____

How often can you commit to doing these exposures?

_____

How will you incorporate them into your daily routine?

_____

_____

_____

Now that you have completed your uncertainty script, continue to play around with it. Reread it ten to twenty times a day, aiming to increase your willingness to be uncertain in any way possible. You may choose to rewrite it and include more triggering material. It is also helpful to record yourself reading your script and listen to the script while engaging in your daily activities. If you feel particularly brave, listen to your recording while engaging in other exposures from chapter 6, particularly exposure to objects, people, events, or sensations that you have avoided because of OCD.

Self-Compassionate ERP Using Acceptance Scripts

Acceptance is an integral part of SC-ERP. Acceptance scripts involve accepting what you do and do not have control over. Acceptance scripts acknowledge that you do not have control of your thoughts, feelings, sensations, images, or urges and that compulsions will not successfully remove the anxiety, uncertainty, and doubt that you experience. Acceptance scripts acknowledge that life is uncertain and that resisting this fact will only cause more suffering. It is important to remember that these scripts are not done to invalidate your pain and your challenges with OCD. Quite the opposite. Acceptance scripts are compassionate, truthful affirmations that can help you lean into your recovery roadblocks and face them with wisdom and compassion.

Step 1: Connect with Your Compassionate Self

Acceptance can often trigger grief, sadness, anger, and anxiety. As you move into writing your first acceptance script, connect with your compassionate self and tend to any pain and suffering that you experience as you anticipate this upcoming exposure.

Putting Your Skills into Practice

Use the space below to reflect on your experience with acceptance. Does the concept of acceptance bring you comfort or discomfort? Do you notice any self-judgment or self-criticism arise as you consider the idea of accepting uncertainty and anxiety in your life?

_____

_____

_____

If any discomfort or self-judgment surfaces, is there a self-compassion meditation or exercise that might connect you to your compassionate self as you move into this exposure?

_____

_____

_____

Step 2: Self-Compassionate ERP

In this script, you will fill in the blanks and also repeat some of the acceptance statements provided. Todd will provide you with an example as you draft your first acceptance script. This exposure will involve you confronting some hard truths about your OCD and will prompt you to change how you move forward with your obsessions and compulsions. Try to be aware of your internal experience as you move through this scripting exercise. Some people report that it becomes easy to fall back into self-criticism and the use of a harsh tone of voice.

Putting Your Skills into Practice

Exposure: Acceptance Script Template

"My name is _____, and I have OCD."

Todd: "My name is Todd, and I have OCD."

"I accept that I will ..." [Insert the uncomfortable, intrusive, repetitive thoughts, images, feelings, sensations, and urges you experience.]

Todd: "I accept that I will have the 'not right' feeling and intrusive thoughts about my future being dismal and heartbreaking."

_____

_____

"I accept that these thoughts, feelings, images, sensations, and urges do not define me and do not disqualify me from treating myself with respect, compassion, and care."

Todd: "I accept that these thoughts, feelings, images, sensations, and urges do not define me and do not disqualify me from treating myself with respect, compassion, and care."

_____

_____

_____

"I accept that my compulsions will only provide me temporary relief from my obsessions and will end up ..." [Insert the consequences of performing compulsions.]

Todd: "I accept that my compulsions will only provide me temporary relief from my obsessions and end up taking me away from the things I value, the people I love, and from living a joyful life. Compulsions always make me feel worse in the long run."

_____

_____

_____

"I accept that being uncertain is the only way to break free of OCD. I accept that I may never know if ..." [Insert your specific fear.]

Todd: "I accept that being uncertain is the only way to break free of OCD. I accept that I may never know if I will be successful or if I will ever feel 'right' again."

_____

_____

_____

Once you have written your acceptance script, read it aloud slowly and clearly as often as you find helpful. Try to really settle into accepting these truths.

RESPONSE PREVENTION

Now that you have written and read your acceptance script, continue to prioritize your response prevention practices. Use the space below to reflect on the prompts provided.

Putting Your Skills into Practice

On a scale of 1 to 10 (with 1 being not willing at all and 10 being very willing), how willing were you to stay in a place of acceptance?

1-------2-------3-------4-------5-------6-------7-------8-------9-------10

Do you have any aversion to practicing acceptance? If so, what struggles are you having?

_____

_____

_____

Did you feel compelled to engage in a compulsion? If so, which ones?

_____

_____

_____

What tools can you use to help as you practice SC-ERP?

_____

_____

_____

Step 3: Nurture Uncertainty and Doubt

Using the space below, reflect on the following questions.

Reflection

Did you say your acceptance script in a kind, nurturing way or in a demanding, directive way?

_____

What self-compassion practices were helpful as you practiced acceptance? What phrases, words, or actions brought you a sense of nurturing?

_____

_____

_____

Step 4: Reflect, Celebrate, and Repeat

In the space below, use the prompts to explore your experience with acceptance scripts: reflect on your progress, celebrate your progress, and plan for future SC-ERP using acceptance scripts.

Reflection

Reflect

On a scale of 1 to 10 (with 1 being not judgmental at all and 10 being highly judgmental and self-critical), how successful were you at not judging yourself negatively or being self-critical during this activity?

1-------2-------3-------4-------5-------6-------7-------8-------9------10

Did you engage in any compulsive behaviors during this exercise? If so, which one? How might you correct this in future ERP?

_____

_____

_____

_____

What got in the way of your willingness to be accepting during this exposure?

_____

_____

_____

Looking back on your SC-ERP, what could you do before, during, and after writing or reading this acceptance script to create a more compassionate experience?

_____

_____

_____

Celebrate

How can you celebrate your successes with this exposure? Is there someone you can share this with? What could you say to yourself that would motivate, support, and encourage you?

_____

_____

_____

Repeat, Repeat, Repeat!

How often can you commit to reading this acceptance script? How will you incorporate them into your daily schedule?

_____

_____

_____

Now that you have written your acceptance script, practice reading it several times throughout the day. Again, you can record your script and listen to the script while engaging in daily activities.

Key Points to Remember

- The more you practice experiencing your intrusive thoughts and subsequent anxiety, the more empowered you will become.

- The goal of scriptwriting is _not_ to make the intrusive thoughts, feelings, sensation, or urges go away. Instead, the goal is to practice having your intrusive thoughts, images, sensations, feelings and urges without engaging in safety-seeking compulsions.

- Scripting is a process, and you should not expect yourself to be perfect or even good at it immediately. Give yourself time and take baby steps.

- If these exposures make you uncomfortable, uncertain, and anxious, _you are on the right path!_ Lean in!

- _It's a beautiful day to do hard things!_

CHAPTER 9

Self-Compassionate Interoceptive Exposures

There will be times when you will find yourself avoiding specific physical sensations within your body. This is common for those who experience panic attacks, sensorimotor obsessions, or any obsession that triggers an uncomfortable physical sensation, such as an increased heart rate, nausea, or dizziness. In these cases, we use what is called "interoceptive exposures" to purposely induce these sensations so you can practice tolerating and willingly allowing them. These exposures often involve a degree of creativity and sometimes silliness to induce the specific sensations. Alex and Todd will walk alongside you as you practice these SC-ERP exercises.

Step 1: Connect with Your Compassionate Self

Before you engage in this exposure, check in with whatever physical sensations you are already feeling. In step 1, your goal is to meet each and every sensation without resistance or judgment. It is entirely normal and okay to struggle with meeting your discomfort with self-compassion. Even the *intention* of being self-compassionate is a wonderful step in the right direction.

Putting Your Skills into Practice

In the space below, write a letter from your compassionate self, sharing how you plan to meet and allow the physical sensations you are feeling and will feel as you engage in this exposure.

Dear Todd,

You are brave for being willing to try these interoceptive exposures. This is not easy work, so take a moment to take pride in what you're doing. Try not to be hard on yourself. Simply observe all of the feelings, sensations, and urges that arise with curiosity and care, and try to be open and willing to allow them to come and go as they please. Never forget that you are stronger than you know. With time, the discomfort of these exposures will rise and fall on their own. Just be gentle with yourself as this happens.

Love, Todd

_____

_____

_____

_____

_____

_____

_____

Step 2: Self-Compassionate ERP

I've provided a list of the most common intrusive sensations and some corresponding interoceptive exposure ideas in the table below. Use it to identify any specific physical sensations you experience intrusively and repetitively. You may also return back to your inventory of intrusive sensations documented in chapter 5. If your particular sensation is not listed in the table below, list it in the empty spaces at the bottom of the table and get creative at finding different ways to induce this sensation. At first, you may want to start slowly and work your way up to more difficult exposures. If you find the listed exposure is not challenging enough, try to find a repetition and intensity that produces your specific feared sensation.

Disclaimer: If you have a history of epilepsy, seizures, fainting, low blood pressure, heart conditions, asthma, or neck or back problems, or if you are pregnant, please consult with your doctor and inform them of the physiological exercise you plan on engaging in. It is advised to get medical clearance before performing any of the below interoceptive exposures.

If you have sensorimotor obsessions and the focus of your obsession is on a particular body part or body sensation, you can practice interoceptive exposures by focusing on your intrusive physical sensation on purpose throughout the day. Set reminders on your phone or leave sticky notes around the house or your workplace to remind you to become aware of the sensation you previously avoided. These reminders will give you the opportunity to purposely tolerate the discomfort of that sensation or awareness while engaging in your daily activities wholeheartedly and compassionately.

Putting Your Skills into Practice

In the table below, put tally marks next the interoceptive exposures you engaged in.

Aversive Sensation	Interoceptive Exposure Options	Completed Tally Marks
Increased heart rate	Run on the spot for one-minute increments. Do twenty pushups (depending on your fitness level). Walk up and down a set of stairs for two minutes (while holding the handrail for safety).	
Tightness in chest	Wrap a bandage tightly around your chest and take a brisk walk for two to five minutes.	
Nausea	Search the internet for videos of people vomiting and watch them for three- to five-minute increments.	
Dizziness or light-headedness	Spin in a chair repeatedly. Hold your breath for ten to thirty seconds. Sit in a chair and put your head between your legs for thirty seconds and then stand up quickly (keeping one hand on something steady, like a table, for safety). Blow a whistle loudly for one minute.	
Derealization or depersonalization	Stand ten inches from a wall and stare for one or two minutes without blinking. Stare at yourself in a mirror without blinking. Stare at a florescent light and then try to read something.	
Sweating	Sit in a hot room, sauna, hot tub, or hot bath. Attend a hot yoga class.	
Trembling or shaking	Drink a cup of strong coffee. Hold weights out in front of your body for one minute. Sit against a wall with no chair for two minutes.	

Aversive Sensation	Interoceptive Exposure Options	Completed Tally Marks
Shortness of breath	Breathe at a fast pace with as much force as you can for one minute. Blow up several balloons in a row. Breathe through a narrow straw for one minute.	
Other:		

Response Prevention

Now that you have practiced your interoceptive exposure, allow the physical sensation to be present, without engaging in safety-seeking compulsions to make it go away. Using the prompts below, reflect on your response prevention practice.

Putting Your Skills into Practice

On a scale of 1 to 10 (with 1 being not willing at all and 10 being very willing), how willing are you to tolerate the sensations you are experiencing?

1-------2-------3-------4-------5-------6-------7-------8-------9-------10

Are there any compulsions you felt compelled to engage in? If so, which ones? How long are you committed to not engaging in these compulsions?

Todd   Because Todd had experienced a severe case of panic attacks, he avoided any activity that induced any panic symptoms. Todd reported that he experienced chest tightness, increased heart rate, and dizziness when having a panic attack. At first, Todd started practicing interoceptive exposures by doing twenty pushups on my office floor to get his heart rate up. After practicing allowing this sensation, Todd then introduced another interoceptive exposure, this time to dizziness. Todd sat in my rotating office chair and spun around quickly thirty to forty times. Todd reported that these two interoceptive exposures did induce the sensations of his panic attack almost exactly, causing him a significant degree of anxiety. Todd practiced performing these two activities, pushups and spinning at varying durations, multiple times per day.

Alex   Alex identified that he avoided any sensation of jitteriness, in fear that he would snap and lose control and harm his innocent students. Alex reported that the last time he had a coffee with a friend, he had a rush of intrusive thoughts about harming his students and his friend, which ended in a severe panic attack. Over the next few weeks, Alex practiced having coffee every morning with his breakfast before school. Alex started by just having one-third of a cup of coffee and worked his way up to then having a large cup each morning. With time, Alex then practiced coupling this interoceptive exposure with his flooding and imaginal scripts before starting his school day.

_____

_____

_____

_____

_____

_____

Step 3: Nurture Anxiety, Uncertainty, and Doubt

As you continue to be uncomfortable, use your self-compassion skills to practice allowing the sensations you are experiencing right now.

Reflection

Using the space below, reflect on the following questions.

Is there a specific self-compassion exercise that helps you hold space for your discomfort instead of pushing it away? How long can you commit to practicing this self-compassion exercise?

_____

_____

_____

_____

Are you using your self-compassion practice to meet and greet your discomfort, or are you using self-compassion to make the discomfort go away? If you answered the latter, how might you adjust your practice to avoid making the sensation go away?

_____

_____

_____

_____

Step 4: Reflect, Celebrate, and Repeat

Congratulations! You completed yet another set of SC-ERP practices. You must be really feeling proud of yourself. If you struggled, please don't give up. Use the below questions to help you troubleshoot what is working and what is not. Remind yourself that it is entirely normal to struggle with these exposures. It will take time, but you will slowly improve with patience and practice. Don't forget to use self-compassion as a catch-all for the emotions that arise as you review your progress. There is no experience self-compassion cannot handle!

Reflection

Reflect

On a scale of 1 to 10 (with 1 being not judgmental at all and 10 being highly judgmental and self-critical), how successful were you at not judging yourself negatively or being self-critical during this exposure?

1-------2-------3-------4-------5-------6-------7-------8-------9-------10

Did you engage in any compulsive behaviors during this exposure? If so, which ones?

_____

_____

What got in the way of your willingness to staying with the physical sensations? What could you do next time to increase your willingness to be uncomfortable instead of engaging in compulsive behaviors?

_____

_____

_____

_____

What could you do before, during, and after these exercises to create a more compassionate experience as you practice interoceptive exposures? Refer back to chapter 3 for a refresh on self-compassion exercises.

_____

_____

_____

Celebrate

How can you celebrate your successes with this exposure? Is there someone safe and supportive you can share this with? What could you say to yourself that would motivate, support, and encourage yourself?

_____

_____

_____

Repeat, Repeat, Repeat!

What could you do next time to make this exposure a little more challenging? How often can you commit to doing these exposures? How will you incorporate them into your day?

_____

_____

_____

Try to incorporate interoceptive exposures into your daily SC-ERP plan as often as you can. The good news is that these exposures do not take up a lot of time, so you can introduce them throughout your day.

Key Points to Remember

- Intrusive sensations can feel really scary, but the more you practice sitting in the discomfort, the more you will learn that you can tolerate them and live your life in their presence.

- The presence of intrusive sensations is not the problem. Our reaction and aversion to them is the problem.

- Don't be afraid to get creative with these exposures. Find new and inventive ways to introduce these sensations into your day as much as you can.

- _It is a beautiful day to do hard things!_

CHAPTER 10

Getting Creative with
Self-Compassionate ERP

Performing exposure and response prevention exercises can be exhausting and sometimes defeating. It can also feel like nothing but work and dread. If this is the case for you, this chapter might put a bit of pep back in your step!

One of the many reasons I love ERP so much compared to other psychological treatment styles is that there are many opportunities for you to make your treatment and your recovery fun. (Yes, you read that right—*fun!*) In this chapter, you will have an opportunity to play around with your obsessions and practice taking the seriousness out of all the thoughts, feelings, sensations, images, and urges you have. With Simone's help, this chapter aims to give yourself permission to have a little fun with your thoughts and create a more playful relationship with your obsessions. As you move through the activities, use this as an opportunity to practice non-judgment and self-compassion. If you enjoy one or all of the activities, try not to get pulled into trying to figure out *why* you enjoyed them. If you do not enjoy them, try not to judge yourself for that. Again, there is no agenda here except to practice staring your fear in the face!

If your first thought is, *I want nothing to do with being playful with my thoughts,* lean in, my dear friend! Reacting to a thought as if it is serious and important will only reinforce that your thoughts are serious and important, making it much stronger and scarier. But responding to your obsessions in a more playful and curious manner can help you break your O-C cycle.

The SC-ERP exercises in this chapter can be used anytime and anywhere as a part of your self-compassionate ERP plan. You may practice them as many times as you like, either going straight to your most challenging obsessions or working your way up from easier obsessions. As you go, be sure to employ *all four steps* of your SC-ERP plan.

And remember, *it's a beautiful day to do hard (and creative) things!*

ERP Sing-Along!

Everyone loves a good sing-along, right? Even if you think your singing skills are atrocious, an ERP sing-along is an excellent way to practice ERP in a playful manner. One of my favorite ERP games for

OCD is the Happy Birthday Obsession Song. It is quite simple. You sing your specific obsession to the melody of the happy birthday song you have been singing since childhood. You simply replace the words of the song, with a phrase describing your obsession. If you need some guidance on how this might sound, you can find a recording of Simone's Happy Birthday Obsession Song on the website for this book (http://www.newharbinger.com/47766).

Simone

"I will kill my pa-tients!" (replacing "happy birthday to you")

"I will kill my pa-tients!" ("happy birthday to you")

"I will kill every single one of them!" ("happy birthday, dear _____")

"I will kill my pa-tients!" ("happy birthday to you")

Putting Your Skills into Practice

In the space below, identify and write the obsession you plan on implementing into the Happy Birthday Obsession Song.

_____

_____

Now, go ahead and try it!

In my career, some of my patients have also courageously created their own lyrics, poems, and spoken words about their obsessions, flooding them with their worst fear coming true. You can have as much fun as you like with this. Don't be afraid to go all out and add dance moves to match your obsessions theme. If you have harm obsessions, add a good karate kick or some of the moves from Michael Jackson's "Thriller." If you have sexual obsessions, add a good twerk or a hand gesture that triggers anxiety, uncertainty, or doubt. If you can't think of anything, try just dancing to your favorite song while replacing the words with your current obsession. I have seen many patients really embrace their obsessions using music and dance, and even though it was overwhelmingly scary and awkward at first, they ended up bursting into fits of laughter by the end of the exposure.

One-Up Game

Another challenging yet fun way to expose yourself to your fear is to play the One-Up Game. This game can be played by yourself, with your therapist, or with family and friends who understand your obsession and symptoms and want to support you in your OCD recovery. The One-Up Game is a helpful exercise if you are struggling to say your specific fear out loud. The rules of the game are quite simple. You start by saying one of your fears aloud. You may choose an easy fear or go directly to a more difficult one. Once you have stated your fear, you or your friend can then follow a more specific thought or a thought that is more triggering.

Simone   Simone and I played the One-Up Game in almost every session once she began practicing SC-ERP. We agreed that no words or phrases were off limits. Below is a script of the One-Up Game Simone and I played to her fear that she will offend God.

Simone: "Offend."

Me: "Offend God."

Simone: "I might offend God."

Me: "I offended God."

Simone: "I offend God, and he never forgives me."

Me: "I offend God, and he hates me."

Simone: "I offend God, and he will not allow me into heaven."

Me: "I offend God, and I go to hell."

Simone: "I offend God, and I go to hell for eternity."

Putting Your Skills into Practice

In the space below, identify what specific obsessions you could use for this exercise.

_____

_____

How you might implement this exercise in your daily routine? Who might you ask to play this game with?

_____

_____

Now go ahead and try it!

Color Your Obsession

Another effective way to expose yourself to your fear is to get creative with the words or phrases that scare you. For this activity, your task is to find one word or phrase that triggers you and write the word in large hollow letters that can be colored in. You can use whatever font you please—block letters or calligraphy, or you can even get fancy and use an online program to create a custom font that feels effective and engaging. Once you have the word down on paper, color it in and really let the word or phrase sink into your being.

Putting Your Skills into Practice

Choose a word that triggers you, and in the space below, write it in hollow letters and color it in. Try to be as creative as you can.

Simone

I AM A SINNER

I am a killer

Draw Your Obsession

A really effective way to expose yourself to the intrusive thoughts and images you have is to practice drawing your obsession on paper. There is no need for talent in this activity, so don't worry about your drawing ability. It's about *what* you draw, not *how* you draw. Put in as much detail and creativity as you like in your drawing. As always, the more detail you can give, and the more you can lean into your fears, the more empowered and confident you will feel in managing your obsessions.

Putting Your Skills into Practice

In the space below, draw a detailed picture of your obsessions coming true. You can reference Simone's drawing below for inspiration and a simple example.

Simone's Exposure Drawing: On one side of a piece of paper, Simone drew a stick figure of herself in the pharmacy, pouring pills into a pill bottle for a patient. She drew the patient standing on the other side of the counter, smiling—happy to be getting the medicine she thinks will help her. On the counter, Simone drew the bottle she had taken the pills from, and drew a skull and crossbones on the label—it's the wrong medicine. On the other side of the paper, she drew her patient's family weeping next to the patient's grave, and then she drew a picture of herself behind bars in prison. Finally, she drew a picture of the devil standing near the jail, waiting to take her down to hell.

Diorama

Another fun and creative way of practicing exposures is to create a diorama of your obsession's worst-case-scenario scene. In this exercise, you can use any materials around the house to make it—cardboard, fabric, paints, play dough, and children's figurines to create the scene of your feared obsession. Do your best to lean into your fear and uncertainty as much as possible, adding more difficult details as you go. You can also practice being mindful and compassionate toward yourself while you are making the diorama, noticing what textures you feel, smells you smell, and so on.

Simone   Simone put a lot of effort into this diorama exposure and created a figurine of herself using clay. Simone embraced her creativity in this exercise by acting out the stories of her scripts inside her diorama to intensify her imaginal scriptwriting exposures. Simone created figurines of pills, pill bottles, her patient, the devil, and other objects and items that triggered her obsessions and compulsions. Simone also took pictures of each scene with her phone so she could look at the diorama during her breaks at the pharmacy, as another way to practice exposing herself to her fear, while practicing response prevention and self-compassion.

Putting Your Skills into Practice

In the space below, identify the details of the diorama you plan to create and set a date in your calendar for when you plan to build it.

_____

_____

In the space below, list the tools and materials you will need to complete this exposure activity.

_____

_____

_____

Setting Reminders

You will find that some days are so busy that you completely forget to do your exposures and your response prevention. In this case, I encourage you to invest in purchasing a pack of sticky notes and leave reminders of your obsession in as many places as you can. You could write your flooding statement (from chapter 7) on as many sticky notes as you can and stick them in your wallet and on your bathroom mirror, refrigerator, steering wheel, and so forth. You may also have some fun by adding emojis or drawings to compliment the reminders. Every time you see it, use this as a cue to practice your imaginal scripts, flooding exposures, interoceptive exposures, or one of the creative ERP games provided in this chapter. You can also create an obsession-related screen saver for your computer or tablet using images and graphics to remind you of your obsessions, giving you the opportunity to practice an exposure or response prevention. Another idea is to set up reminder alerts on your smartphone that will tell you when it is time to practice exposures—or just an alert that will remind you of your obsession. The goal with reminders is to be sure that you have many opportunities to stare your fear right in the face throughout each day.

Putting Your Skills into Practice

In the space below, identify which reminder exercises you will implement into your daily routine. Be as specific as you can.

Simone

- "Set reminders on my smartphone each day at 9 a.m., 11 a.m., and 3 p.m. that say, 'Don't forget, you might kill your patient today!' "

- "Put an image of a skull on my screensaver to remind me to do flooding exposures related to my moral and religious obsessions."

_____

_____

Now go ahead and put these reminders in place!

CHAPTER 11

Managing Strong Emotions During ERP with Self-Compassion

All humans experience intense, turbulent emotions. However, for some people, these waves of emotion are more frequent and can lead to painful self-criticism and self-hatred. This is especially true for many individuals with OCD. Experiencing relentless, repetitive obsessions all day long and feeling entirely controlled by your compulsions often results in intense emotions such as panic, shame, guilt, anger, sadness, and disgust, just to name a few.

It is essential to understand that there is no such thing as a "wrong" or "bad" emotion and that each emotion serves an important role in your life. With the assistance of self-compassion, you can learn to meet each and every emotion, even the really strong and painful ones, with tenderness instead of resistance. The practice of self-compassion will help you manage the strong emotions that may arise as you engage in ERP. While self-compassion will not prevent or stop a strong emotion from arising, it will help you to wade through the emotion in a way that does not create more problems (second arrows). By creating a respectful and compassionate space for these emotions, you can also learn to trust your ability to ride out any difficult experience.

General Coping Skills for Strong Emotions

Below are some general coping skills to help you manage whatever intense emotions arise. After these general skills, you will have an opportunity to learn specific tools to help manage the most common strong emotions experienced during ERP. Todd and Simone will be the case studies for this chapter and will share their practices managing strong emotions.

Name the Emotion

Before you can manage an emotion, you must first name it. Sometimes when emotions are strong, particularly anxiety, it becomes difficult to identify the other emotions that are surfacing. When you become aware of strong emotions arising, first ask yourself, "What emotion am I feeling right now?" During ERP, people with OCD often experience strong waves of anger, guilt, shame, and sadness.

Sometimes identifying these emotions and saying, "I am feeling X right now," can help you step back from the emotion and learn to respond to it with compassion instead of with judgment and resistance. If you are struggling to find a name for the emotion you feel, you may use the list below. Another great idea is to do an internet search for "emotions chart." There are many fun and helpful graphics of faces to help you identify what emotion it is that you are feeling.

Putting Your Skills into Practice

In the list below, reflect and highlight or circle the emotion(s) you are feeling.

Acceptance	Envy	Panic
Affection	Fear	Pride
Amazement	Gloom	Regret
Anger	Grief	Remorse
Apprehension	Guilt	Resentment
Astonishment	Happiness	Revulsion
Contrition	Hostility	Sadness
Depression	Irritability	Shame
Despair	Joy	Shock
Disgust	Loneliness	Sorrow
Dread	Melancholy	Surprise
Embarrassment	Nervousness	Trust

Validate Your Experience

Once you have named your emotion, then be sure to validate yourself and the strong emotion you are feeling. There is no emotion that you "should not" feel. It is healthy to have all of the emotions, and all emotions are valid, even when they are strong and don't make sense to other people. You might benefit by saying to yourself, "I am feeling X, and that is okay. Everyone feels this emotion sometimes. I am not weak or wrong for feeling this way."

Go Through Emotions, Not Around Emotions

Many people make the mistake of trying to run away from emotions. In the field of psychology, we often acknowledge that you cannot selectively avoid emotions. If you numb the difficult emotions, you will most likely find that you numb the positive, joyful emotions also. A helpful coping skill when feeling strong emotions is to go *through* the emotion, not around it. Allow the emotion to wash over you like a wave. Remember, they call them "feelings" because you are supposed to *feel* them, not push them away. As you willingly feel your emotion, engage in something you enjoy or participate in the daily activities you would typically engage in, had this emotion not arisen. While you feel this strong emotion, try to fully engage in whatever activity you are doing, and use it as an opportunity to practice having strong emotions without letting the emotion stop you from doing the things you love. If a strong emotion arises while practicing ERP, try to lean into the emotion while practicing response prevention. Remind yourself that you can handle many emotions at the same time. You can tolerate uncertainty and fear *while* you feel angry or sad or ashamed or guilty. This might feel impossible, but it isn't. You already have everything you need to do this courageous and empowering work.

Meet Your Emotion with Self-Compassion

No matter how strong the emotion is, try to lean into it and make lots of space for it to rise and fall on its own. If the emotion becomes particularly painful and powerful, lean into it with every ounce of self-compassion you can muster up. The more difficult the emotion, the more self-compassion you offer yourself. You can return to any of the self-compassion tools you learned in this workbook if you are struggling.

Stay Present: Every Emotion Is Temporary

No emotion lasts forever. Even if it feels like it will break you, try to remind yourself that emotions cannot permanently hurt you. They are all temporary. When you experience a strong emotion, recognize that this emotion is like a wave in the ocean. It will rise, but inevitably it will fall, and with time, patience, and acceptance, you can ride it out.

Coach Yourself Through the Emotion

Sometimes it can be helpful to coach yourself through an emotion, similar to how you coach yourself through an exposure using your compassionate self. If a strong emotion arises, use your kind coach voice to guide you through this difficult time. Remember, a kind coach would use language that is encouraging, supportive, and warm. You might want to say, "Right now, I am noticing a strong wave of shame. Just because I feel shame does not mean I have anything to be ashamed of. I am going to allow it to be there and be as kind and calm as I can. This feeling is temporary, and it will pass. I am going to finish up that project in the backyard. I am not going to let shame stop me from doing the things I love." You might also want to coach yourself by using encouraging statements such as "Keep going. You have got this!" or "Look at how you are feeling your feelings without engaging in compulsions or being self-critical! Good for you!"

Putting Your Skills into Practice

Using your kind coach to guide you, write a statement or two that might help you manage this emotion in the space below.

_____

_____

_____

_____

Key Points to Remember

Useful practices to use when managing strong emotions.

- Name the Emotion

- Validate Your Experience

- Go Through Emotions, Not Around Emotions

- Meet Your Emotion with Self-Compassion

- Stay Present: Every Emotion Is Temporary

- Coach Yourself Through the Emotion

Specific Tools for Common Strong Emotions

Now that we've covered the general skills for coping with strong emotions, I'll give you some special tools that will help you address a few of the most common and powerful emotions—panic, anger, guilt, shame, and sadness.

Managing Panic with Self-Compassion

Let's be honest. One of the most torturous experiences in the world is panic. A panic attack is a combination of different intense anxiety symptoms. If your anxiety levels are at a 10 out of 10, you are likely having a panic attack. Common panic symptoms include increased heart rate, a tight chest, dizziness, stomachaches, derealization, depersonalization, light-headedness, shortness of breath, vision issues, tingling, and many more. Similar to any other experience of anxiety, your instincts will naturally want you to run away from the sensations and events of a panic attack. The first thing to know is that a panic attack will not hurt you or do any kind of permanent damage. The other thing you must remember about panic is that the more you try to make your panic go away, the more likely you are to have higher degrees of anxiety and panic. The more you fight it, the more it controls you. In addition to the tools at the beginning of this chapter, another trick to managing panic is to radically allow whatever sensations of panic you feel by saying, "Bring it on!" The panic will rise and fall on its own, and your only job is to not rush through it. Ride it out like it is a wave in the ocean. If it goes high, go high with it, and don't fight it. If it goes low, don't cling to it to try to make it stay low. Your job is to compassionately commit to riding the waves. I know this might sound counterintuitive—and even completely preposterous—but believe me when I say that standing up tall and leaning into panic will be the most empowering thing you do, next to facing your obsessions head-on during ERP. You may find it helpful to practice some compassionate breathing while experiencing panic. The goal of incorporating compassionate breathing is not to make the panic go away but to give you a focal point for your attention. As you notice and allow panic symptoms, try to bring your attention to the rise and fall of your breath.

Putting Your Skills into Practice

When you are experiencing panic, experiment with these skills and then answer the journal prompts below.

- Bring your attention to your breath and try to find a steady rhythm as your chest rises and falls.

- As you notice physical discomfort (dizziness or a stomachache or a tight chest) arise in your body, practice acknowledging each area of discomfort and saying yes to it. You may also experiment with saying, for example, "You are welcome here, dizziness."

- Try to unclench your hands and jaw and relax your shoulders and stomach as you breathe.

- Talk with your panic as if it were a separate person: "Panic, I am cool with you being here. Bring it on!"

- Bring your attention to your surroundings while you let your panic rise and fall on its own. Look for shapes and colors, listen for noises, or become aware of the different scents in the space you are located.

Reflection

On a scale of 1 to 10 (with 1 being not willing at all and 10 being very willing), how willing am I to allow the discomfort that accompanies this panic?

1-------2-------3-------4-------5-------6-------7-------8-------9------10

Of the skills provided in the list above, which one allowed me to ride out the panic attack most easily, without resisting or fighting the discomfort I felt?

_____

_____

_____

Anger and Self-Compassion

Just like all emotions, anger is an important and necessary emotion. Anger is a protective emotion that shows up when you feel threatened or when something is wrong. Anger moves us toward the perceived problem instead of away from it, and it propels us toward eradicating the threat. Anger also arises when you—or someone you care about—are exposed to injustice or are criticized. It can also arise when you feel overwhelmed.

At an early age, many of us were taught that anger is not an appropriate emotion and that we must not let anger get the best of us. In some cases, we were taught that anger is "bad" or "wrong." But suppressing anger goes against our human instincts. When we do not allow ourselves to feel anger or do not use it to move toward a resolving action, we may engage in unhelpful behaviors such as rumination, resentment, negative self-assessment, or self-blame. It is also possible that our attempt to suppress the anger will fail, and anger will overwhelm us in a furious outburst.

Reflection

Below is a list of the most common reasons people with OCD feel anger. Reflect on your own experience and mark off the ones that resonate with you.

☐ I feel angry that I have OCD.

☐ I feel angry because my intrusive thoughts are relentless, and I am unable to control them.

☐ I feel angry because OCD takes me away from the life I want to live.

☐ I feel angry because I get stuck performing compulsions that I do not want to perform.

☐ I feel angry when people judge me as "lazy" and "weak" for doing compulsions.

☐ I feel angry when people comment on how I am handling my anxiety.

☐ I am angry when people say "I am so OCD" about something trivial, when they clearly have no idea how hard it is to have OCD.

☐ I am angry because my past doctors and therapists did not help me and gave me incorrect advice.

☐ I am angry that I have to do ERP to get better.

☐ I feel angry because no one understands what it is like to have OCD.

☐ Other: _____

If you checked one or all of these points, you are definitely not alone. The main thing to remember is that you are never bad or wrong for feeling angry. You have every right to feel angry, and I encourage you to give yourself permission to just feel the anger when it arises. As discussed above, anger is an emotion whose function is to propel us toward change or resolution. Practicing self-compassionate ERP is the solution to many of the items on the above checklist. Self-compassionate ERP will help you learn how to tolerate your intrusive thoughts, feelings, images, sensations, and urges without engaging in compulsive safety behaviors, including negative self-talk and self-punishment.

When you feel anger, try to go through this feeling, not around it, as mentioned earlier in this chapter. As you allow anger to rise and fall at its own pace, bring your attention to your breath, do some compassionate breathing exercises, or perform any other self-compassion practices that resonate with you. Use your compassionate self to guide you as you wade through this powerful but important emotion. If helpful, you may choose to effectively communicate your anger with a loved one or a friend to help you troubleshoot ways to manage the stressor or adversity that is causing your anger.

Reflection

Use the space below to reflect on what comes up for you when experiencing anger.

Using the compassionate wisdom inside me, what is this anger trying to tell me?

_____

_____

_____

Is there another emotion (or more than one) underneath this anger? If so, can you name it (or them)?

_____

Can I be kind and tender toward my anger? What tools might be helpful to me right now?

_____

_____

_____

_____

_____

Are there ways I can take compassionate responsibility for this anger? What can I do to heal this anger without engaging in compulsions or other behaviors that take me away from my recovery or well-being?

_____

_____

Something to Consider

If you experience certain obsessions—like harm, scrupulous, pedophilia, or other sexual obsessions—you may fear that feeling anger will make you snap and do something unforgivable. In this case, common compulsions include anger avoidance, reassurance seeking, and ruminative analysis about the real motive or intention of one's anger. If this is the case for you, you will need to practice intentionally inducing anger (as an exposure) and tolerating the anxiety and uncertainty that this emotion produces. While this might feel like the scariest thing to you, I still encourage you to lean in and practice it.

Managing Guilt with Self-Compassion

Guilt is an important and helpful emotion. Guilt may arise when you have broken a rule, hurt someone, or made a mistake. You may also feel guilt when you see others facing adversity and hardship that you don't. When there is a problem, guilt may arise, propelling you to identify whether you have played a role in creating the problem and then pushing you to troubleshoot ways to solve the problem and to prevent anything similar from happening again in the future. Ultimately, guilt's job is to propel us toward making amends for our wrongdoings.

People with OCD often feel extreme degrees of guilt, most of which is highly unwarranted and disproportionate to their actions. This is called "undeserved guilt." Undeserved guilt is commonly the direct outcome of unrealistic and perfectionistic expectations of oneself. A heightened sense of responsibility, called "hyper-responsibility," will also cause undeserved guilt. If you have unrealistic expectations of yourself or feel hyper-responsible for events that are outside your control, it is likely that your feelings of guilt are never-ending. It is also likely that your guilt is accompanied with painful degrees of self-criticism, extreme frustration, and rumination, because your expectations of yourself are unrealistic and unachievable.

Reflection

Below is a checklist of some of the common reasons people with OCD feel guilt. Reflect on your own experience with guilt and check off the points that resonate with you.

I feel guilty because:

☐ I have intrusive thoughts, feelings, images, urges, or sensations that I deem "wrong," "bad," "inappropriate," or "immoral."

☐ I expect myself to manage my obsessions and compulsions better.

☐ I experience arousal in situations I deem "inappropriate" or "wrong." (This is common with sexual obsessions.)

☐ I experience urges to harm a loved one, colleague, or friend. (This is common with harm, scrupulous, relationship, or sexual obsessions.)

☐ I experience "false memory" obsessions and cannot be sure if those memories are real or not.

☐ I did not "give enough" or "worry enough." (This is common for those who experience hyper-responsibility.)

☐ My OCD has impacted my loved ones.

☐ My OCD treatment has required the financial resources of my loved ones.

☐ Other people's difficulties seem greater or different than mine.

☐ I require myself to feel guilty, proving that I am a good, moral human being.

☐ I feel guilt intrusively and spontaneously. It just shows up when it wants!

☐ Other: _____

☐ Other: _____

If you checked off any of the points in this checklist—or even a lot of them—please remember, just because you *feel* guilt, does not mean you *are* guilty and deserve to be punished. For people with OCD, guilt will often present itself as an obsession (intrusive feeling), making you feel like you urgently need to solve all of your "wrongdoings." Through practicing SC-ERP, your job is to allow the feeling of guilt and go about your day, bringing guilt along for the ride. If you are going to the grocery store, or if you are trying to finish that one work project, take guilt along with you. It may be present, but that doesn't mean you have to give it your attention.

It is also important to remember that your obsessions and compulsions do not make you a terrible person and do not warrant a marathon of self-criticism. As you move through your OCD recovery, you will need to recognize wholeheartedly that it is not your fault that you have OCD. Let me repeat this. *It is not your fault that you have OCD.* You did not ask for this, and you do not deserve it.

If you feel guilt for things that you did in the past, recognize that you were doing the best you could with the resources you had at that time. Maybe you didn't have the tools you needed at that moment to respond in the way you wanted. Or perhaps you didn't know what to do or how to respond because you were flooded with anxiety and uncertainty. Maybe you knew what to do, but you had not yet had the practice of standing up to your OCD, and at that moment, you performed compulsions out of pure desperation. Whatever happened at that moment, you were doing the best you could with what you had.

Ruminating and beating yourself up for past events will not motivate you to act differently next time you are in that position. In fact, quite the opposite is true. In addition, trying to mentally solve whether or not you should feel guilty—or if your guilt is warranted—is also ineffective and is a compulsion. The most compassionate and effective thing you can do when you feel strong waves of guilt is to radically accept yourself, along with whatever did or did not happen in the past, and then practice being uncertain while giving yourself the self-compassion you need. This is *not* letting yourself off the hook. This is responding wisely, effectively, and compassionately. Chances are that you have kept yourself on the hook for long enough, and that didn't seem to bear a good outcome, so let's try using only kindness and warmth when guilt arises.

If you find that you are constantly having to manage guilt in your life, I have created a new set of rules that you may use to set more realistic expectations of yourself. I encourage you to embrace each and every one of them with warmth and compassion.

Key Points to Remember

- Perfection does not exist, and I cannot expect myself to be perfect in any area of my life.

- I will have days when I do well and days when I don't.

- There is no such thing as a good or bad thought or image, a good or bad feeling, a good or bad sensation, or a good or bad urge.

- There is no such thing as perfection.

- Recovery is not linear. Recovery includes ups and downs.

- My worth has nothing to do with another person's opinion of me.

- Having OCD or another mental illness does not determine my worth.

- "Should" and "must" are opinions, not facts.

- I am allowed to make mistakes. All humans make mistakes. When I make a mistake, I will commit to not ruminating about it.

When Guilt and Anxiety Serve as
a Form of Reassurance

There may be times where your guilt and anxiety serve as a form of reassurance. This is especially common for those with harm, moral, religious, relationship, or sexual obsessions.

Simone   When distributing medications at the pharmacy, Simone would often feel a deep sense of guilt and anxiety because of her intrusive thoughts and urges about harming her patients. While Simone hated feeling guilty and anxious all the time at work, she did notice that the presence of these emotions often comforted and reassured her. Simone said, "If I feel guilty about my obsession, that proves that I do not want to poison my patients, right?"

When experiencing guilt and anxiety, try to become aware of moments when you are trying to use these emotions as reassurance or proof that your fears will not come true. Instead, make space for the uncertainty you feel and try not to fight it. And tend to your uncertainty, anxiety, and other emotions with loving-kindness and non-judgment.

Self-Compassion and Shame

Sometimes, instead of feeling guilt, you might experience shame. While guilt is the emotion you experience when you feel that you have done something wrong or unwanted, shame is the emotional experience that you *are* wrong and unwanted. Shame is a powerful and painful emotion that all humans feel to different degrees. When you feel shame, you feel profoundly flawed and broken—it impacts your self-identity and self-worth. When you feel shame, you will feel that you are "not enough" and, therefore, could be or should be discarded and abandoned or punished.

Reflection

People with OCD often experience a high degree of shame. Use the checklist below to identify what triggers shame in you.

Shame arises in me when:

☐ Society stigmatizes OCD and other mental illnesses.

☐ I have intrusive thoughts that I deem as "wrong" or "bad."

☐ I have intrusive images that I deem as "wrong" or "bad."

☐ I have intrusive urges that I deem as "wrong" or "bad."

☐ I have intrusive sensations (such as arousal) that I deem as "wrong" or "bad."

☐ I have feelings (such as anger, fear, guilt, or irritability) that I deem as "wrong" or "bad."

☐ I engage in compulsions that have impacted myself or others.

☐ I compare myself with others who are not struggling with similar challenges.

☐ Other people judge me or place their expectations on me.

☐ Other _____

☐ Other _____

Before we move on to some additional tools to use with shame, I first want to highlight the impact shame has on those who have obsessions seen as "taboo." These obsessions include sexual obsessions, harm obsessions, scrupulous obsessions, moral obsessions, perinatal obsessions, bestiality obsessions, sodomy obsessions, and sexual-orientation obsessions. Given that these topics are already taboo in our general culture to one extent or another, it makes total sense that you struggle immensely with shame if you experience these obsessions day in and day out.

It is crucial to remember that your thoughts do not define you. Just because you have thoughts that feel shameful does not mean you have anything to be ashamed of. This is an excellent opportunity to practice the skill of non-judgment, the skill of recognizing that there is no such thing as a "bad" thought or a "good" thought. The same goes for intrusive sensations, urges, images, and feelings.

When shame arises, name it by gently saying, "This is the voice of shame" or "Shame just showed up." This will help you to first disengage with shame's messaging and then move into self-compassion faster. As mentioned before, the messaging of shame usually revolves around the idea that you are not worthy of love and will soon be abandoned. Your job is to recognize that shame has shown up and do your best to reframe the messaging by reminding yourself that just because you feel shame, that does not mean you have anything to be ashamed of. You are worthy of love, no matter what you think, feel, or do.

When shame arises, it is also helpful to recognize that you are not alone in this struggle. Millions of people are going through similar struggles, thinking the same thoughts. Consider self-compassion to be the most healing medicine for shame when it arises. Try to meet your shame with tenderness, recognizing that everyone, even those who do not have OCD, have strange, intrusive thoughts that are sometimes taboo. It might be helpful to also acknowledge that everyone is struggling with something. While the people you know might not have OCD, I can guarantee that they carry some burden that brings up shame for them too. If possible, find a safe and supportive person and talk with them about experiences with OCD and the shame that you feel. You might find that while they don't understand your specific experience, they understand the experience of shame and understand how painful shame can be. You might even find they will also benefit significantly from learning how to lean into fear and practice self-compassion skills. If you don't feel comfortable talking with a family member or friend about your shame, reach out to a trained mental health professional or a support group in your area and seek support in that way. Shame thrives on secrecy, so if you can practice talking with someone about it, you might find that shame has less power over you.

My patients and clients have found compassionate letter writing to be incredibly helpful in managing shame. As well as writing letters to yourself, you may also find it helpful to write a letter directly to your shame, as if it was an external entity. Writing letters can help you to practice using your compassionate voice for when you experience shame in real time. Below is an example of a compassionate letter written by Todd.

Dear Shame,

I see that you are here with me again, and that is okay. I am going to be very gentle with you. No longer am I going to allow you to say hurtful words to me. I have OCD, but I am not bad or wrong or horrible for this. Also, shame, I know you keep telling me not to tell anyone about my thoughts and not to ask for help, but I deserve to get treatment for my OCD. You are welcome to show up any time along the way, but I am choosing to treat myself gently and compassionately from now on.

Love,

Todd.

Putting Your Skills into Practice

Using the space below, write a letter to the shame that you experience from you.

_____

_____

_____

_____

_____

_____

_____

Self-Compassion and Sadness

Sadness is the emotion that follows a challenge, a hardship, or a hurtful interaction. Sadness alerts us when our needs, or someone else's needs, are not being met, and it draws us toward connection. When we feel sad, we naturally feel compelled to ask for closeness, commonality, and others' assistance. Ultimately, sadness is a sign that we need support and care. People with OCD often become overwhelmed with sadness because of how much OCD has taken from them.

Reflection

Using the checklist below, note the points that resonate with you.

I feel sad because:

☐   OCD has taken me away from doing the things I enjoy.

☐   OCD has tormented me with intrusive thoughts, feelings, sensations, images, and urges.

☐   OCD has caused me to miss important events.

☐   OCD has made me question my identity.

☐   Exposure and response prevention is hard and exhausting.

☐   I feel alone, like no one understands what it is like to have OCD.

☐   Having high levels of anxiety and uncertainty is incredibly painful.

☐   Other: _____

☐   Other: _____

As discussed at the beginning of this chapter, it is crucial that you first validate your experience of sadness instead of pushing it away or trying to hide it. You might also need to practice not judging yourself for your sadness and, instead, meet your sadness with a sense of inquiry.

Reflection

If you are struggling with sadness, use the prompts below to reflect on it.

What do you need right now?

_____

_____

_____

How can you soothe yourself (in a non-compulsive way) as you feel this sadness?

_____

_____

_____

Is there someone you could ask to sit with you as you feel this sadness? (Note: If you don't feel comfortable talking with anyone, that is entirely okay.)

_____

Which self-compassion practice would help soothe my sadness right now?

_____

_____

_____

There may be times when sadness becomes so overpowering that you feel like you can barely move your body. If this is the case for you, focus on doing small tasks that bring you a sense of satisfaction or joy. Slowly and patiently, engage in an activity that helps you compassionately manage as your sadness passes through you. Remind yourself that sadness, like all emotions, is temporary, and there is no need to push them away. The sadder you feel, the kinder and more compassionate you will need to be toward yourself. Do whatever you can to kindly and respectfully hold space for the sadness you are experiencing. Also, remember that you must not compare your pain with another person's pain. Your sadness about having OCD is equally valid as anyone else's struggles.

Also, please note that if this feeling of sadness becomes chronic, pervasive, and spreads across most or all of the areas of your life, you might be experiencing depression. Depression is a mental illness that includes many other emotional problems, such as difficulty sleeping, loss of energy, loss of pleasure, and loss of concentration. If you think you might be depressed, reach out to a mental health provider or a medical health provider in your area.

PART THREE

Recovery and Beyond

Creating Your Most Compassionate Life

Dear courageous and resilient one,

If you have progressed this far into the workbook, chances are you are exhausted. Most individuals with OCD report that ERP is the most challenging thing they have ever done—but also the most empowering thing they have ever done. When we are exhausted, our natural inclination is to collapse and give up. The exhaustion feels never-ending.

Now, before you give up, try wrapping yourself and your exhaustion in the largest metaphorical self-compassion blanket you can imagine and place your attention on replenishing your energy stores.

Take some time to honor your exhaustion. Rest! Practice some of the self-care activities given in this chapter. But then, get right back up and take another step—whether that is a big step or a teeny, tiny step—toward taking your life back from OCD.

Sending you love and strength,

Kimberley

CHAPTER 12

Self-Compassionate ERP Practices for Long-Term Recovery

This chapter talks about the long game, helps you integrate self-compassionate ERP as a fundamental part of your life, and sets up a long-term recovery plan. But before we do that, let's talk about what "recovery" from OCD really looks like.

What Is Recovery from OCD?

As much as I would love to end this book with a miraculous story about how you, after practicing self-compassionate ERP, will go on to live a life free from all of your anxiety and obsessions, I am going to keep it real for you. Recovery from OCD is not eliminating your intrusive thoughts, images, urges, sensations, and feelings; nor is it the removal of anxiety, uncertainty, and doubt. Instead, recovery from OCD involves courageously *living the life* you want to live instead of letting OCD tell you what to do all day long. Recovery from OCD means that *while* you experience obsessions, anxiety, and uncertainty, you live your life as compassionately and as fully as you can, without using safety-seeking compulsions to remove or reduce your anxiety, uncertainty, and doubt. Of course, no one is perfect at this, and that is totally okay. The thing to remember is that recovery is possible.

"Recovery" also involves your giving yourself some slack for the bumps along the way. It is important to understand that OCD treatment is not a linear process, and everyone's recovery looks different. You will need to pace yourself and be prepared for it to be messy. You will have good days, and you will have really hard days. You will have days when your exposures are easy and other days when they feel impossible and make you collapse from exhaustion. *All* of this is completely normal. All you need to do is get back up and keep going!

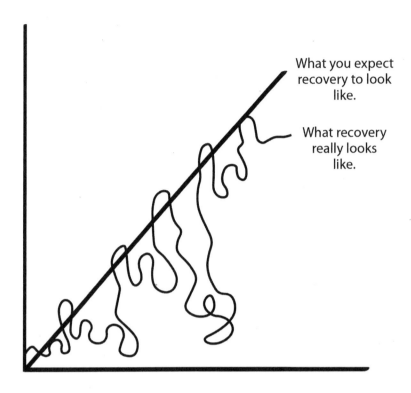

Figure: What OCD Recovery Really Looks Like

Recovery from OCD also requires not just behavioral changes but mindset shifts as well. Some of these shifts will happen naturally as you continue to practice SC-ERP, whereas others might need continuous reminders. These mindset shifts will involve changing how you respond to your obsessions and compulsions and how you expect your life to look with OCD.

Reflection

Below are some examples of Alex's old mindset before treatment compared to his new recovery mindset. These mindset shifts were *crucial* to Alex's long-term recovery. I strongly encourage you to embrace these mindset shifts in every area of your life. Then, using the table below, add in any additional mindset shifts you need to remember as you continue on your OCD journey.

Old Mindset	Recovery Mindset
"I am not supposed to have these thoughts."	"No matter what, I am going to allow these thoughts."
"My obsessions make me a bad person."	"My obsessions do not define who I am and what kind of person I am."
"I cannot do this anymore."	"I can do this for just one more day."
"I will get better as soon as I stop these obsessions."	"Recovery involves focusing on the reduction and illumination of compulsions, not obsessions."
"I am an idiot for having OCD."	"People with OCD are badasses. They are as worthy as anyone else. I can live a fulfilled life with this diagnosis."
"My anxiety sucks, and I hate it."	"My anxiety is not the problem. How I respond to my anxiety is the problem."
"I will do these exposures because they will make my anxiety go away."	"I am going to do my exposures, not to reduce anxiety, but to learn that I can tolerate the anxiety."
"One day, OCD will go away, and then I can live my life."	"OCD does not simply disappear after treatment. Having OCD is something I have to learn to manage. I can still live my life fully, even with OCD."
"I will do my exposures as soon as my anxiety lowers a little."	"I will do my exposures now. The more willing I am to be anxious, the more I will get out of this exposure."
"This fear and uncertainty must mean something."	"Trying to figure out what it means will only feed me back into the O-C cycle. I will be uncertain instead."
"I will face that fear tomorrow."	"Today is a beautiful day to do hard things."
"I am not strong enough to do ERP."	"I will try anyway."

Old Mindset	Recovery Mindset

Now, I acknowledge that these mindset changes may take a while to embrace. These are not concepts that you can adopt simply by reading them once. Please go easy on yourself as you wade through this process. Long-term recovery from OCD takes compassion, time, patience, and *lots* and *lots* of practice. Feel free to refer back to this workbook as much as you need. I have crafted this workbook to be a helpful resource at every step of your recovery. (What an honor!)

Developing Long-Term Exposure Practices

Once you have worked your way through your ERP Challenge List and practiced all the exposures given in this workbook, I strongly encourage you to continue practicing self-compassionate ERP for at least forty-five to ninety minutes per day. Ideally, you will maintain this routine for as long as you can, being sure to adjust your exposures and your response prevention as your obsessions and compulsions wax and wane. Over time, you may find that the content of your obsessions and compulsions change. This is not uncommon at all. Do your best not to catastrophize on days when they are loud and persistent. Go back to earlier chapters in this workbook and apply the same self-compassionate ERP steps to the new obsessions and compulsions.

If you notice a sudden increase in obsessions or safety-seeking compulsions, you will have to increase your self-compassionate ERP practices in those areas. As you become more familiar with what works for you specifically, you will be able to gauge the correct frequency, duration, and intensity of your exposures. Usually, the more intense an obsession, the more intentional and engaged you will need to be with your exposures and response prevention.

At What Point Can I Stop Doing Exposures?

Todd   Todd had been practicing ERP for some time now, and he was beginning to really get his life back from OCD. Todd had returned to his social activities and no longer needed his parents to accommodate his OCD. Todd was able to perform the tasks asked of him without engaging in compulsions. He did sometimes catch himself engaging in mental compulsions (or other compulsions). Still, overall, he felt confident again, and he was less distressed about the intrusive thoughts that he was having. Todd asked, "At what point can I stop doing my exposures?"

Even if your symptoms have reduced, I still encourage you to always make it a point to seek out the things that scare you so you can practice your self-compassion and mindfulness skills on a daily basis.

If you are consistently able to tolerate your intrusive thoughts, feelings, images, sensations, and urges without engaging in safety-seeking compulsions, you can start to reduce the frequency and duration of your exposures slowly. You could start by lowering the frequency of your exposures to only every other day, and then, if you are successful at maintaining your skills, you may try reducing the frequency and duration more and more over time.

Long-Term Self-Compassionate Response Prevention

Your ability to resist the urge to engage in safety-seeking compulsions will determine who is in the driver's seat of your life: you or OCD. While it is okay to slowly reduce your daily exposure practices slightly (depending on your symptoms), you must do your best to hold your ground and not return back to engaging in compulsions. Response prevention is crucial to your long-term recovery. Once you have eliminated a compulsion from your daily life, do your best to maintain that progress. Employ your self-compassion and mindfulness skills as much as you can to maintain your response-prevention skills.

If you notice an obsession return (or if you experience a new obsession), do your best to immediately identify what compulsions you feel the urge to engage in and return back to all four steps of your self-compassionate ERP plan. Those steps are there to support you in every stage of your recovery, and there is no shame in going back and creating a whole new ERP Challenge List for a new (or returned) obsession.

Long-Term Self-Compassion Practices

Todd   Todd was transitioning down to seeing me only once a month and was successfully continuing with his ERP and daily self-compassion practices on his own. Todd reported that he was feeling much better about himself now. He said, "It's strange. I still have the thoughts, but they bother me so much less now. I am wondering if I need to be doing these self-compassion practices daily."

Even when life is going well, and your anxiety is calm, I still encourage you to continue a strong and consistent self-compassion practice. I always say that having a solid self-compassion practice is like a superpower that you can take with you throughout life, no matter what happens in your life. You can use it anytime and anywhere, and it costs absolutely nothing. (Bargain!) Right now, as I am writing this, we are eight months into the COVID-19 pandemic, and I cannot tell you how many times I have used these skills to help me manage the strong emotions and hardships that I have felt. When life gets hard, whether related to OCD or not, practice self-compassion unconditionally. Unconditional self-compassion means that there is never a day where you do not deserve—or require—meeting your pain and suffering with self-compassion. Remember, the practice of self-compassion is a practice of equality. No one is disqualified. Self-compassion is not conditional, and it not something you practice only when times are difficult.

Key Points to Remember

If you are anything like me, you never loved math. However, here is some basic math that you might be able to get on board with …

- *You* + the most upsetting intrusive thought = Deserving of Love and Self-Compassion

- *You* + a strong intrusive feeling = Deserving of Love and Self-Compassion

- *You* + the strongest, most concerning urge = Deserving of Love and Self-Compassion

- *You* + the most violent intrusive image = Deserving of Love and Self-Compassion

- *You* + the strangest intrusive sensation = Deserving of Love and Self-Compassion

- *You* + making giant mistakes during recovery = Deserving of Love and Self-Compassion

- *You* + being terrible at self-compassion = Deserving of Love and Self-Compassion

- *You* + having a mental illness = Deserving of Love and Self-Compassion

- *You* = Deserving of Love and Self-Compassion

Reflection

Are there any other "equations" that you want to add to this list? If so, put them below. Try your best to create your own "self-compassionate equation" to represent specific areas where you struggle to practice self-compassion.

_____

_____

_____

Self-Care Is the Ultimate Self-Compassion Practice

The concept of self-care has been greatly misunderstood in our society. When we speak of self-care, many people think of bubble baths, expensive candles, and luxurious spa days. While these are some examples of self-care, these activities are often not sustainable and can detract from the true definition of what self-care actually is. Self-care is an activity that is done to preserve and restore your mental or physical health. Brushing your teeth is an example of self-care. You brush and floss your teeth not because it makes your life fabulous, but to preserve the wellness of your gums and teeth. You go for a yearly check-up with your doctor not because this brings you tremendous joy and pleasure, but because you value keeping your body healthy. Self-care is not always an act of pleasure (though it can be). It is an intentional practice that you engage in to take care of your wellness.

Unfortunately, our society places a high degree of attention on the importance of medical and physical health without considering the importance of taking care of our mental health. Societal norms have prioritized beauty over rest, productivity over peace of mind, and other people's opinions of us over our opinion of ourselves. In this chapter, we will aim toward prioritizing our entire being, including our mental health, by creating your personal self-care plan. It is also likely that your obsessions and compulsions have taken many of your self-care practices away from you. Use this as an opportunity to *take back your life from OCD* and find a self-care routine that is both helpful and realistic.

The practice of self-care requires asking yourself, "What do I need right now?" Self-compassion involves being willing to honor your needs and wishes at a time and pace that feels right to you. Self-care is different for everyone and will require you to practice a large degree of non-judgment. You might need to rely on some of your self-compassion or mindfulness practices as you create a self-care plan that is helpful for you.

Simone   When Simone and I discussed self-care, I asked her, "Take a few minutes and think of three to five things you could do this week to restore your mental and physical health."

After a few minutes, Simone said, "I would really benefit from going to bed earlier so I can get a little more sleep. I will be sure to do that tonight. I would also love to take one weekend just for me. No people. No events. Maybe even paint my nails. I have not done that in so long. But … it all seems a little self-centered."

I responded by asking her why she judged herself for wanting alone time but was so nonjudgmental about her need for additional sleep. She was able to identify that she struggles to allow herself to have alone time because she feels a high level of responsibility to please her family and friends. I asked Simone to question her self-judgment for herself needing alone time for self-care. She was able to recognize that she was prioritizing other people's needs over her own. This did not mean that Simone needed to stop seeing her friends and family completely. It simply meant that she would listen to her body and take a day off here and there to rest and restore her energy so she could keep moving through her ERP Challenge List.

You might find that your idea of self-care is completely different from Simone's. As you move throughout your recovery, check in with yourself consistently, and ask what you need to feel mentally revitalized and stay motivated to continue with SC-ERP.

Reflection

Below is a list of possible self-care activities. You will notice that many of them are free or require very little money. This is intended to help you set up a self-care plan that is maintainable. Use the check boxes and check the self-care activities that you feel would complement your SC-ERP practices. If you are struggling to identify self-care activities that sound enjoyable, simply check off five to ten activities that you are curious about. Once again, self-care does not need to center around providing immense pleasure. Instead, it might simply be an opportunity to practice your self-compassion and response-prevention skills.

Please note that these self-care activities should not be used to resist your anxiety or uncertainty. If you find yourself using self-care compulsively, return back to the four steps of SC-ERP and practice willingly allowing your discomfort.

- ☐ Take a bath.
- ☐ Call a friend.
- ☐ Take some time alone.
- ☐ Nap.
- ☐ Take a walk outside, in nature.
- ☐ Play with a pet.
- ☐ Watch a lighthearted show.
- ☐ Set limits and boundaries with people who take up your energy.
- ☐ Set an alarm to ensure that you wake up at your desired time.
- ☐ Drink more water.
- ☐ Say no to things you do not want to do.
- ☐ Say yes to things that scare you but will make you feel connected with others.
- ☐ Learn a new hobby.
- ☐ Buy a weighted blanket.
- ☐ Give yourself a manicure.
- ☐ Go to a religious service of your choice.
- ☐ Watch funny videos on the internet.
- ☐ Plan a reward for doing hard exposures.
- ☐ Plan to meet up with a friend who supports you.
- ☐ Set boundaries with people who use unkind words.
- ☐ Go to the bathroom when you need to.
- ☐ Begin a meditation practice.
- ☐ Stretch your body.
- ☐ Dance alone in your pajamas.
- ☐ Order in a lovely meal.
- ☐ Ask a friend to pick up your kids from school so you can do an exposure.
- ☐ Tell your friends and family that you no longer want them to reassure you.
- ☐ Buy a lovely skin cream to moisturize your skin.
- ☐ Set limits with how much work you do after hours.
- ☐ Go to bed at the same time each day.
- ☐ Diffuse essential oils or burn a candle of your preference.
- ☐ Take time away from your phone every day.
- ☐ Say no to events that do not enrich your life.
- ☐ Reach out to a therapist or support person when you are struggling to do this work alone.
- ☐ Allow other people to have their own strong emotions without taking responsibility for them.
- ☐ Give yourself permission to have whatever feelings you experience.
- ☐ Limit your exposure to social media or the news.
- ☐ Offer yourself compliments and encouragement.
- ☐ Wear comfy clothing and shoes.
- ☐ Stop criticizing your body.

Now that you have identified what self-care activities interest you, reflect on the below questions.

When can you schedule these self-care activities?

_____

_____

_____

_____

Are there any products or items you need to practice these self-care activities? If so, where will you get these items? What budget will you set for self-care?

_____

_____

What roadblocks might get in the way of your practicing these self-care activities?

_____

_____

How can you plan for these roadblocks?

_____

_____

Gather Your OCD Team!

You deserve help and support. Having OCD can feel incredibly isolating, so please give yourself permission to reach out and get help in whatever way feels right to you. Just knowing you are not alone and that other people are going through similar experiences can be incredibly healing and can give you the motivation to keep going.

Fortunately, there are many online resources that can offer support and a sense of community as you continue on your OCD journey. Try doing an internet search for online groups, forums, and organizations in your local area that can offer you support and kinship. You may also find it helpful to join an OCD support group where you can share and discuss the challenges of having OCD. You can also find excellent resources online that can offer excellent psychoeducation about OCD:

- The OCD Stories Podcast: https://theocdstories.com.

- My podcast (Your Anxiety Toolkit Podcast): https://kimberleyquinlan-lmft.com/podcast-blog.

- The International OCD Foundation: https://iocdf.org.

- The OCD Gamechangers: https://ocdgamechangers.com.

- The website of therapist Shala Nicely, who works with OCD and related disorders: https://www.shalanicely.com.

- Made of Millions (whose mission is to change the way people see mental illness): https://www.madeofmillions.com.

- The Anxiety and Depression Association of America: https://adaa.org.

- If you have a coexisting eating disorder, go to the website of the National Eating Disorders Association for education and resources: https://www.nationaleatingdisorders.org.

- If you have a coexisting body-focused repetitive behavior, the TLC Foundation for Body-Focused Repetitive Behaviors offers support and resources: https://www.bfrb.org.

While I have done my best to cover every possible angle of exposure and response prevention, self-compassion, and mindfulness, you may find that you require a higher level of care. If this is the case, I strongly encourage you to reach out to a trained OCD therapist. Below are a few excellent options for additional support for OCD.

- Go to the website of the IOCDF (https://iocdf.org) and use the search page to find a mental health professional who is trained to use exposure and response prevention. Do not be afraid to ask where they got their training and how much experience they have.

- Find a peer support counselor who can support you and help with motivation and psychoeducation while you practice SC-ERP.

- If you need more intensive support, again, use the IOCDF directory and inquire about the options for intensive outpatient services or intensive inpatient facilities in your area. The IOCDF works tirelessly to stay up to date on the options for more intensive OCD treatment. If you struggle with substance abuse or another coexisting disorder, let them know when you inquire, and they can direct you to facilities and centers that will accommodate your needs.

CHAPTER 13

OCD and Trauma, Grief, and Loss

We can be thankful for the many researchers and clinicians who developed exposure and response prevention. ERP has allowed people with OCD to learn how to resist engaging in safety-seeking compulsions and how to effectively respond to their obsessions when they arise. However, as mentioned throughout this book, long-term healing is not just addressing one's symptoms of OCD. We must look at the whole person (you) and address the psychological impact of having OCD. This book would not be complete without acknowledging the experience of trauma, grief, and loss that results from being tormented by terrifying intrusive thoughts, images, sensations, feelings, and urges. The experience of trauma, grief, and loss is a common by-product of OCD. It is also important that we address how the onset of OCD can be particularly traumatic and how OCD can fracture your identity, sense of self, and mental health.

In this chapter, you will learn how Tanya and Alex used self-compassion to tend to the trauma, grief, and loss related to their experience of OCD. You will also have an opportunity to put these skills into practice and acknowledge the trauma, grief, and loss that have been part of your experience.

Having OCD Is a Form of Trauma

Alex   As Alex neared the end of completing the tasks on his ERP Challenge List, he was able to return back to work and could get through an entire day without being overly consumed by his obsessions. This was a huge accomplishment, as at one point, Alex had been unable to even leave the house in fear that he would harm someone. Even though Alex was feeling much better, he still reported a consistent hypervigilance and was still having recurring memories of himself curled up in a ball, crying, and being terrorized by his intrusive thoughts and images. Alex also reported that he could not stop thinking about the many times when he got stuck in compulsions, unable to stop them, and felt like he was out of control. As Alex reported these symptoms, he would squint and tense up his body, as if he was reexperiencing his most horrifying moments of OCD. Alex said, "Even though I am feeling so much better about my obsessions and compulsions, the memories of those times haunt me."

As a mental health professional that has treated OCD for over a decade, I, without a doubt, believe that having these severe repetitive and intrusive obsessions and compulsions over a period of time can result in a trauma response. Similar to being held hostage at gunpoint by a robber, OCD has the ability to create what feels like a life-threatening moment all day long. This causes the person with OCD to respond in ways that reinforce the danger alert, recreating the experience of terror over and over again.

Alex   When I suggested to Alex that having OCD can be considered a form of trauma, he denied this concept entirely. Alex responded, "This is not trauma. 'Trauma' is a word used when someone has been sexually or physically assaulted, has been held hostage, or was a prisoner of war. This is just my stupid brain making drama out of every little thing. I just want to finish ERP and forget this whole thing ever happened."

I was taken aback by Alex's response to my suggestion. Alex's self-criticism and denial of his own suffering concerned me, as it showed just how judgmental he was of his experience with these symptoms and how much he invalidated his own suffering. Alex's response also revealed that he was still internally stigmatizing himself for having OCD.

I responded, "Alex, I wonder if you could think of the term 'trauma' on a spectrum? On one end of the spectrum is someone with zero symptoms of trauma, and on the other end would be those who meet the criteria for the diagnosis of post-traumatic stress disorder (PTSD). People with PTSD typically have witnessed or experienced a serious event that threatened their sense of safety and well-being, causing them to experience emotional responses such as flashbacks, strained relationships, hypervigilance, depression, and isolation. While you might not meet all the criteria for PTSD, you do land somewhere on the trauma spectrum, which means you deserve the time and space to address and heal all that you have experienced since the onset of your OCD. While you may not have been involved in a violent car accident or witnessed the death of another person, you did go through the traumatic event of having terrorizing obsessions and feeling so stuck in your compulsions. I wonder if you could validate that experience instead of avoiding or denying the impact it had on you as a human being?" With this explanation, Alex was able to acknowledge and validate the influence OCD had on his life.

Self-Compassion Tools for Trauma

As you move through your recovery, it is important that you too acknowledge any indications of trauma, no matter where you are on the spectrum of trauma. Denying your experiences can lead to multiple secondary struggles, such as isolating behaviors, avoidant behaviors, and high levels of shame and depression, just to name a few. Once you acknowledge your own emotional experience and trauma response, you must validate the pain and suffering you endured throughout your experience of having

OCD. Try to compassionately validate just how hard it was (and still is) for you. Try to take time each day to recognize how hard it was for you to feel that much anxiety, uncertainty, and doubt for as long as you did (and possibly still do).

Putting Your Skills into Practice

Connect with the compassionate self that lives within you, and in the space below, offer yourself a few validating statements about your experience of having OCD and how hard it was for you.

Alex: "Having OCD was and still can be very hard for me. There were times when I felt I could not go on because the thoughts were so tormenting. The voice of OCD was harsh and made me feel terrible about myself."

_____

_____

_____

In the space below, complete this sentence. "It makes complete sense that I feel ..." [Insert a validating statement about your suffering.]

Alex: "It makes complete sense that I feel hypervigilant and overwhelmed. Most people would feel this exact way if they went through what I have been through."

_____

_____

_____

What self-compassion skills and practices might help you when you notice yourself struggling with traumatic memories of having intrusive, repetitive thoughts, images, sensations, feelings, and urges?

Alex: "I think what I need most is validation instead of denying or disallowing the fact that I went through an incredibly hard period. I also think that I need to slow down when I have these intrusive memories and really bring myself back into the present. I need to practice not suppressing these memories and instead be compassionate toward them. I often get taken away with my thoughts, and when I have them, they feel incredibly real. When I have intrusive memories about times when I was struggling with OCD, I will stop, put my hand on my heart, and bring my attention to my surroundings. I will look for shapes, colors, smells, different textures, and aspects of everything around me."

_____

_____

_____

_____

_____

_____

_____

Sometimes, the traumatic memories and feelings will come back strongly, while other times, you might find that they are consistent and live just under your awareness. This is completely normal and nothing to be alarmed by. As the memories and images return, try to meet them with self-compassion, just like you would any other intrusive, repetitive thoughts or images that you have. If you notice increased or persistent symptoms of trauma; if you are experiencing symptoms of PTSD, such as flashbacks, nightmares, trouble sleeping, difficulty concentrating; or if you are struggling to function because of any of these symptoms, please reach out to a PTSD specialist who is knowledgeable about OCD and exposure and response prevention.

Grief and Loss

Grief is the deep, painful emotional experience of sorrow that follows a loss. This loss might include the death of a loved one or the loss of a relationship, past event, or one's identity. Grief is intense and much more painful than sadness. Grief includes despair and mourning, in addition to the emotion of sadness and many other painful emotions. People with OCD often have a lot to grieve, and this grief can sometimes feel unbearable.

Tanya   Tanya was struggling with completing her ERP work. Tanya reported, "Every time I do an exposure in which I plan to spend time with Julie, and whenever I read my scripts, I get overwhelmed with grief and anger. It reminds me of all of the time I wasted doing compulsions and obsessing over my sexual orientation or our relationship. I mean—I have lost hundreds of hours to OCD, and I just can't let it go. I hate myself for this. I have missed countless moments with Julie. I have missed important events, my family's birthdays, weddings, baby showers, all because of OCD. Even if I was there physically, I wasn't really there. I was preoccupied with my obsessions and stuck trying to solve everything. I just cannot get over the fact that those times are gone forever. It's unforgivable." Tanya sobbed.

If you resonate with Tanya's story, you are definitely not alone. I rarely have a client with OCD who does not need to address the grief that accompanies having OCD at some point in their recovery. OCD can take away the things you love and strips you of your own sense of self and your self-identity.

When you notice grief showing up in your body, try to meet and tend to whatever suffering you feel. Try not to compare your loss with other people's loss. You deserve to grieve the time, energy, and peace of mind that OCD took from you. It is not your fault you have OCD, and it is not your fault that you have intrusive thoughts, images, sensations, feelings, and urges. If anyone else were in your exact position, they would have responded similarly, engaging in compulsive safety-seeking behaviors and wanting to run away from the anxiety, uncertainty, and doubt that they felt. Try to validate yourself for everything you have been through and give yourself ample time to feel your emotions. Remember, all emotions are valid and deserve to be felt. As each emotion rises and falls, place your intention of being kind and compassionate toward yourself and the present emotion.

The Stages of Grief

Author and psychiatrist Elisabeth Kübler-Ross outlined the five states of grief in her book *On Death and Dying* (1970) to help people understand the grief process and the different emotions that are commonly felt:

- denial

- anger

- bargaining

- depression

- acceptance

It is important to recognize that you may not experience all of these stages or in this specific order. You might find that there are times when your grief is well managed and does not require a lot of your attention, while at other times, your grief might be strong and require you to slow down and tend to it compassionately and mindfully. I hope that exploring these stages will validate and normalize any grief you might be feeling and emphasize that there is no "right" way to grieve. Every stage is a normal, healthy response to grief and loss. Let's take a deep dive into the stages of grief!

DENIAL AND OCD

According to Kübler-Ross, *denial,* the first stage of grief, is the experience of denying the suffering you are experiencing. For someone with OCD, this includes denying the things you have lost because of OCD. Sometimes, people with OCD struggle to acknowledge how much pain they are in or how much their obsessions and compulsions have impacted their life (and their loved ones' lives), because it is just too painful to acknowledge so much loss at one time. This is totally understandable. However, over time, this resistance just prolongs their pain and grief and, in many cases, delays their OCD recovery.

If you find yourself denying or avoiding the impact OCD has had on your life, reach out to a safe, caring person (or a mental health professional) who can sit with you and support you as you begin to wade through the loss you feel. As you allow whatever feelings to arise, gently offer yourself some words or gestures of compassion, reminding yourself that there is no emotional pain you cannot tolerate, especially if you do so in a compassionate way. Remember, having OCD is not your fault. You may also benefit by going back to chapter 4 and reviewing your roadblocks to self-compassion.

ANGER AND OCD

There are many reasons you might feel anger when it comes to having OCD. At times, you might find that anger becomes so powerful that you feel like it will never go away. This is normal, and I encourage you to give anger permission to rise and fall on its own. Try not to push it away. As anger arises, try not to engage in self-criticism or self-punishment. Simply acknowledge it, and nurture yourself with every ounce of your being. If you struggle to allow anger, return to chapter 11 for more in-depth instruction on managing and utilizing anger using self-compassion.

BARGAINING AND OCD

Bargaining, the third stage of grief, involves the process of trying to reconcile why the event happened or trying to figure out how one could have prevented a loss in the past.

Tanya   Tanya was struggling with the bargaining stage of grief. Tanya would sometimes lie awake for hours at night going over and over why she got OCD and what she could have done to prevent it. "If I never had thoughts about men, this would never have happened. I could have stopped all of this from happening. If I only had known that this was OCD, I could have gotten better faster. Had I done something different, maybe this would never have happened."

This is what bargaining sounds like. Bargaining usually involves a lot of hindsight, and as they say, hindsight is 20/20. It does not take into account that you were doing the best you could with what you had and that having OCD is not your fault. If you find yourself in the bargaining state, first acknowledge, "I am bargaining. This is a normal part of the grief process," and then try to use one of your self-compassion exercises or skills to help you hold space for the emotions that you are experiencing instead of ruminating about how you could have prevented it, as this can become compulsive. You may also experience a painful degree of guilt and self-blame during this stage of grief.

DEPRESSION AND OCD

Depression, the fourth stage of grief, can be described as the experience of being stuck in a thick, heavy fog. Depression often involves feelings such as hopelessness, helplessness, and worthlessness. Common symptoms of depression include restlessness, trouble sleeping (or sleeping too much), lack of pleasure or enjoyment in activities that usually bring you joy, difficulty eating or concentrating, and physical distress such as stomachaches and headaches. Many people with OCD experience depression, not only as a part of their grieving process, but also as a result of feeling so controlled and trapped by their obsessions and compulsions. Symptoms of depression sometimes include thoughts of suicide (thoughts that do not make one anxious or uncertain, unlike suicidal obsessions). If you are experiencing depression with suicidal thoughts, please reach out to your medical doctor or mental health professional or go to your local emergency room.

ACCEPTANCE AND OCD

Acceptance, the fifth stage of the grief process, is where you come to accept what has happened to you and accept yourself for how you handled the situation. For someone with OCD, acceptance acknowledges that it was never your fault that you had OCD and that you did the best you could with what you had at the time. Acceptance is also acknowledging that your suffering is a part of being a human. While life would have been much easier had you not had OCD, acceptance involves accepting the past, without judgment, comparison, or criticism.

BUT WAIT! THERE'S ONE MORE STAGE

David Kessler, an author and clinician, added one more stage to the grief process. In his book, *Finding Meaning: The Sixth Stage of Grief* (2019), Kessler explained that people who are grieving experience pressure from society to move on and forget their grief. These pressures and expectations interfere with people's healing and create self-criticism. Instead, a person might find meaning in what they have been through by turning their pain into some kind of purpose. Kessler calls this the "finding meaning" stage of grief. This stage is not required in order to move through your grief process. However, some people find that it helps to turn what was a painful experience into something positive or something that gives meaning to the experience.

Tanya   Toward the end of treatment, Tanya was able (most of the time) to be accepting of herself, her obsessions, and everything she had endured throughout her history with OCD. I shared with Tanya how many people with OCD turn their pain into purpose by educating others about OCD—sharing their experience with others—so they feel less alone and can possibly help others who are suffering. Others find meaning by becoming an advocate for mental health rights. When I broached the idea of finding meaning out of her OCD, Tanya reported that she felt anger rise in her body at this suggestion. I was so impressed with Tanya's honesty.

Tanya shared, "I am not able to think about OCD in that way just yet. OCD nearly ruined my entire life. I cannot see how I could find meaning out of such an awful experience."

I acknowledged Tanya's feelings about this, and I was very clear that the "finding meaning" step is optional. Tanya continued with her treatment, placing a heavy emphasis on practicing self-compassion whenever her anger, sadness, grief, or loss arose.

At Tanya's last session with me, she handed me a letter and said, "I know some people turn their pain into purpose by educating and advocating, but I am not that kind of person. Instead, I have written a letter, and I am giving you permission to share it with anyone you think might need to hear these words. This is my way of "turning my pain into purpose."

With Tanya's permission, I am concluding *The Self-Compassion Workbook for OCD* not with a letter from me, but a letter from Tanya. Tanya is a warrior. She struggled very much throughout treatment, but she persevered, and she took her life back from OCD. Here is her letter to you, dear friend! May you be kind to yourself at every single stage of your recovery.

Tanya's letter to *you*.

Dear friend with OCD,

My name is Tanya, and I have OCD. My OCD nearly destroyed my entire life. If you have OCD, I know your pain, and you are not alone, dear friend. I know what it is like to feel like you have been knocked down a thousand times and that you do not have what it takes to get up one more time. I know the anxiety, uncertainty, and suffering you are enduring. I know what it is like to have no hope and no faith.

But here are a few things that I want to share that you might not know just yet. You see, today is my last day of weekly therapy with Kimberley, and I am now moving toward managing OCD on my own. I have my life back now, and I am currently working toward maintaining all that I have learned and practiced.

Here is what I now know:

You are not broken. You were never broken.

Your obsessions do not define who you are. They are stories that your mind tells you. If you can learn to let them simply be here, you will learn to coexist with them.

You can get better. I know this seems impossible right now, but I promise it is true. I didn't believe it either, and here I am.

ERP is so freaking hard you will want to scream many times. This is entirely okay. Go ahead and scream if you like. And then, keep going. There will be days where you want to crawl into bed and cry for days. That is okay too. Have a really good cry and then stand up and keep going.

The anxiety and uncertainty you feel will not hurt you or kill you. This was a big lesson for me and is one I have to work on every day. Practice allowing the discomfort to pass and be as kind as possible while the pain rises and falls within you.

Last one. You are enough. Having OCD will make you think you are not as worthy as others, and this is a huge lie. OCD will also try to convince you that you are not worthy of being loved, and that too is a big fat lie. You are worthy. You are enough. You are strong. Do not give up on yourself.

Love, Tanya

Acknowledgments

Dear courageous reader, thank *you* for trusting me with your recovery journey. You made the decision to stare fear right in the eyes and that is the most remarkable act of courage, resilience, and self-love.

I am proud to say that from day one, this workbook was crafted with compassion being the highest priority. Behind me stood a force of love, support, and encouragement. This workbook would not have come together if it was not for the kindheartedness and support of the following people.

Thank you to Wendy, my acquisitions editor, who somehow believed that I could put my passion onto paper and create this workbook. A huge thank you to Caleb Beckwith and Jennifer Eastman, my editors, for being patient with me and providing such helpful guidance through multiple meltdowns and rewrites.

To my gorgeous husband, thank you for unconditionally supporting me every single day. You are my rock, and I am so grateful for you. You patiently sat with me and listened while I experienced *all* of the emotions as I wrote this book. I love you! To the wisest and most courageous person I know, Shala Nicely, thank you for being my daily dose of encouragement, direction, and inspiration. Thank you to my beautiful Mum for tirelessly reading each chapter and finding "the loveliest word," and for drawing the most adorable smiley faces next to the sentences you loved. Thank you to Jon Hershfield for writing such a beautiful forward for this book. You have been a wonderful mentor to me, and I am so grateful for you. Thank you to Fay and Lisa, my therapists, for holding space for me throughout some of my most difficult times.

Thank you to each and every one of my clients for teaching me everything I know about courage. Being witness to your trials, bravery, and badassery has made me a better therapist, mother, and human.

Lastly, thank you to the following people for your continuous support, contribution, and advice. You were always one text away, and I love each and every one of you: Michelle Massi, Stacey Kuhl Wochner, Sonia Greaven, Brennan Rinehimer, Reid Wilson, Ethan Smith, Chrissie Hodges, Alegra Kastens, Allison Stimpson, Jessica Serber, Nathalie Rutherford, Nicole Pickering, and Natalie Abrahami.

References

Brach, T. 2019. *Radical Compassion: Learning to Love Yourself and Your World with the Practice of RAIN*. Penguin Life.

Gilbert, P. 2010. "Training Our Minds in, with, and for Compassion: An Introduction to Concepts and Compassion-Focused Exercises." https://www.getselfhelp.co.uk/docs/gilbert-compassion-handout.pdf.

Gilbert, P., and Choden. 2014. *Mindful Compassion: How the Science of Compassion Can Help You Understand Your Emotions, Live in the Present, and Connect Deeply with Others*. Oakland, CA: New Harbinger.

Kessler, D. 2019. *Finding Meaning*. New York: Scribner.

Kübler-Ross, E. 1970. *On Death and Dying*. New York: Collier Books/Macmillan.

Neely, M. E., D. L. Schallert, S. S. Mohammed, R. M. Roberts, Y. Chen. 2009. "Self-Kindness When Facing Stress: The Role of Self-Compassion, Goal Regulation, and Support in College Students' Well-Being." *Motivation and Emotion* 33: 88–97.

Neff, K. D. 2012. "The Science of Self-Compassion." In *Compassion and Wisdom in Psychotherapy*, edited by C. K. Germer and R. D. Siegel. New York: Guilford Press.

Neff, K. D., and C. K. Germer. 2018. *The Mindful Self-Compassion Workbook: A Proven Way to Accept Yourself, Find Inner Strength, and Thrive*. New York: Guilford Press.

Norman L. J., S. F. Taylor, Y. Liu, J. Radua, Y. Chye, S. J. De Wit, et al. 2019. "Error Processing and Inhibitory Control in Obsessive-Compulsive Disorder: A Meta-Analysis Using Statistical Parametric Maps." *Biological Psychiatry* 85, no. 9: 713–25. doi: 10.1016/j.biopsych.2018.11.010.

Rector, N. A., R. M. Bagby, Z. V. Segal, R. T. Joffe, and A. Levitt. 2000. "Self-Criticism and Dependency in Depressed Patients Treated with Cognitive Therapy or Pharmacotherapy." *Cognitive Therapy and Research* 24, no. 5: 571–84.

Rockliff, H., P. Gilbert, K. McEwan, S. Lightman, and D. Glover. 2008. "A Pilot Exploration of Heart Rate Variability and Salivary Cortisol Responses to Compassion-Focused Imagery." *Clinical Neuropsychiatry: Journal of Treatment Evaluation* 5, no. 3: 132–39.

Simon D., N. Adler, C. Kaufmann, and N. Kathmann. 2014. "Amygdala Hyperactivation During Symptom Provocation in Obsessive-Compulsive Disorder and Its Modulation by Distraction." *NeuroImage: Clinical* 4: 549–57.

Sugiura, Y., and B. Fisak. 2019. "Inflated Responsibility in Worry and Obsessive Thinking." *International Journal of Cognitive Therapy* 12, no. 2: 97–108. https://doi.org/10.1007/s41811 -019-00041-x.

Tolin D. F., J. S. Abramowitz, A. Przeworski, and E. B. Foa. 2000. "Thought Suppression in Obsessive-Compulsive Disorder." *Behaviour Research and Therapy* 40, no. 11: 1255–74.

Trompetter, H. R., E. Kleine, E. T. de Bohlmeijer. 2016. "Why Does Positive Mental Health Buffer Against Psychopathology? An Exploratory Study on Self-Compassion as a Resilience Mechanism and Adaptive Emotion Regulation Strategy." *Cognitive Therapy and Research* 41, no. 3: pp. 459–468.

Warren, R., E. Smeets, and K. Neff. 2016. "Self-Criticism and Self-Compassion: Risk and Resilience: Being Compassionate to Oneself Is Associated with Emotional Resilience and Psychological Well-Being." *Current Psychiatry* 15, no. 12: 18–32.

Wegner, D. M., D. J. Schneider, S. Carter, and T. White. 1987. "Paradoxical Effects of Thought Suppression." *Journal of Personality and Social Psychology* 53: 5–13.

Wetterneck, C. T., E. B. Lee, A. H. Smith, J. M. Hart. 2013. "Courage, Self-Compassion, and Values in Obsessive-Compulsive Disorder." *Journal of Contextual Behavioral Science* 2, no. 3–4: 68–73.

Williams, J. G., S. K. Stark, and E. E. Foster. 2008. "Start Today or the Very Last Day? The Relationships Among Self-Compassion, Motivation, and Procrastination." *American Journal of Psychological Research* 4, no. 1: 37–44.

Kimberley Quinlan, LMFT, is a psychotherapist in private practice specializing in the treatment of obsessive-compulsive disorder (OCD) and related disorders. She has been practicing meditation and mindfulness for many years, and has a special interest in the integration of mindfulness and self-compassion principles with cognitive behavioral therapy (CBT) for OCD, anxiety disorders, and eating disorders. Kimberley is host of the *Your Anxiety Toolkit* podcast, and founder of www.cbtschool.com—an online psychoeducation platform for OCD, anxiety disorders, and body-focused repetitive behaviors (BFRBs). Quinlan is known for her vibrant and mindful approach to mental health issues, and is an expert presenter and support group facilitator for various conferences worldwide. She has been featured in many world-renowned and prestigious media outlets, including the *Los Angeles Times*, *The Wall Street Journal*, and *The Washington Post*; and has consulted on various mental health issues for programs such as ABC's *20/20*.

Foreword writer Jon Hershfield, MFT, is a psychotherapist specializing in the treatment of obsessive-compulsive disorder (OCD), and is director of The Center for OCD and Anxiety at Sheppard Pratt in Towson, MD. He is author of *Overcoming Harm OCD*, *The OCD Workbook for Teens*, and *When a Family Member Has OCD*, and coauthor of *The Mindfulness Workbook for OCD* and *Everyday Mindfulness for OCD*.

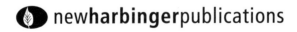

MORE BOOKS from
NEW HARBINGER PUBLICATIONS

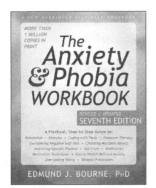
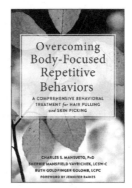
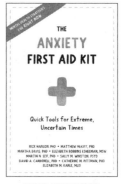
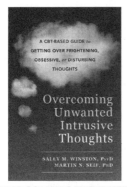
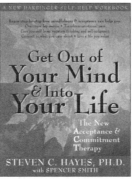
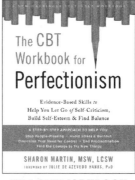

Did you know there are **free tools** you can download for this book?

Free tools are things like **worksheets**, **guided meditation exercises**, and **more** that will help you get the most out of your book.

You can download free tools for this book—whether you bought or borrowed it, in any format, from any source—from the New Harbinger website. All you need is a NewHarbinger.com account. Just use the URL provided in this book to view the free tools that are available for it. Then, click on the "download" button for the free tool you want, and follow the prompts that appear to log in to your NewHarbinger.com account and download the material.

You can also save the free tools for this book to your **Free Tools Library** so you can access them again anytime, just by logging in to your account! Just look for this button on the book's free tools page.

+ Save this to my free tools library

If you need help accessing or downloading free tools, visit **newharbinger.com/faq** or contact us at **customerservice@newharbinger.com**.